To Cleo Davis,
With best wishes
for good health.

Robert Bingham, M.D.

FIGHT BACK AGAINST ARTHRITIS

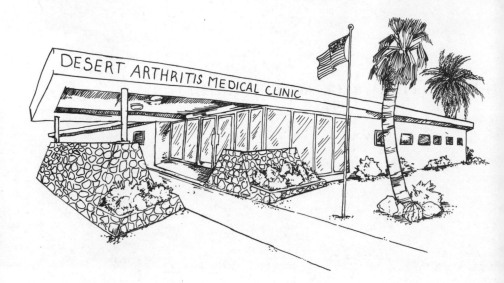

FIGHT BACK AGAINST ARTHRITIS

by

Robert Bingham, M. D.

Medical Director, Desert Arthritis Medical Clinic

Desert Hot Springs, California

Illustrated by Ann Bingham Freeman

Copyright © 1984 by Robert Bingham, M.D.
Published By
Desert Arthritis Medical Clinic
13-630 Mountain View Road
Desert Hot Springs, CA 92240
ISBN: 0-930703-00-6
Library of Congress No. 84-71312

TABLE OF CONTENTS

Dedication

*To my dear wife, Charlotte, who for
almost fifty years has helped me with her
love and loyalty.*

PREFACE

Some mystical force, or should I say spiritual influence, seemed to demand that this book be written. Except for the mechanical steps of typing and dictation the manuscript seemed to write itself. It filled my mind, and the words poured out in a stream of information on arthritis, filling page after page and chapter after chapter. While on my summer vacation I would frequently awaken at three o'clock in the morning with an inspiration. Then I would compose paragraph after paragraph before I could return to sleep again.

Finally the book was finished. This is the first edition. As medical progress continues and the available knowledge about arthritis increases it will be periodically revised.

In an important way the book is different from any other published on arthritis. It features an health oriented approach including combinations of effective treatments, long neglected or forgotten, together with new and innovative approaches to arthritis therapy. These have been gathered from the work and publications of many authorities, combined here for the first time in book form. It includes much that is original, treatments that are different, and new developments regarding the causes of arthritis. Most important are reports and information regarding discoveries that bring hope of "remissions" and even "permanent improvement" for some of the most severe and resistant forms of rheumatoid arthritis.

The wisdom of this book includes experiences gleaned from many years of medical practice in a desert health resort town which is blessed with natural hot mineral waters. For over fifty years, since this natural resource was discovered by Cabot Yerxa, arthritis patients from all parts of the United States, Canada and Mexico have found relief from their aches and pains in the warm, dry desert climate and the therapeutic pools.

This treatment program,which has been successful for so many patients, is a combination of the art and science of medicine. It originated in a free clinic for crippled children, many with juvenile rheumatoid arthritis. What was so helpful for them has proved just as useful in restoring health and strength to adults suffering with arthritis and rheumatism. This is the story that must be told.

The ARTHRITIS PROGRAM was developed with the medical knowledge and contributions of many physicians and biological scientists, M.D.'s and Ph.D's. These include Joseph C. Risser for natural foods and exercise; Francis Pottenger Jr. for advocating certified raw milk; Michael Walsh for the first diet analyses; Bernard A. Bellew for the arthritis vaccine; Johnathon Wright choosing arthritis as a goal of natural methods; Weston A. Price for his pioneer studies of native peoples; John W.Yale, Jr. for basic research on the use of the Yucca plant extract as a food supplement for arthritis patients; Linus Pauling for his advocacy of Vitamin C; the Shute brothers and their use of Vitamin E; J. I. Rodale for "PREVENTION" magazine; Lowell M. Somers for his discovery of "Esterene"; and especially the late Roger Wyburn-Mason for his life's work on the role of amoebae in rheumatoid disease and the drugs which bring improvement and remissions.

The book is written for patients who have arthritis and rheumatism who wish to help themselves, those who will choose to FIGHT BACK AGAINST ARTHRITIS. There are many who now suffer, believing that there is no possible way to get any better. There are many thousands who are dependent on their families for care. The majority of patients cannot afford the time and money to come to the desert area for treatment. This book will be extremely useful to patients who have not improved or recovered with other methods of care.

The book is written for physicians who are seeking improved and alternative therapies for patients who do not respond to conventional drugs and who are fearful of the stronger medications such as gold, penicillamine and the corticosteriods.

The book will tell you how you can help yourself and how you can furnish information to your physician so that he can duplicate these results.

At the DESERT ARTHRITIS MEDICAL Clinic we call this method the ARTHRITIS PROGRAM. The emphasis is on the *patient* more than on the *disease*. It restores the patient to good health, rather than just supplying the patient medicine to reduce symptoms without seeking and removing the *causes,* wherever possible.

One of our discoveries is that *a large number of patients suffer from more than one type of arthritis,* both osteoarthritis and osteoporosis for example. The medicines they have been taking for the one disease may be making the other gradually worse. There is no drug which does not have side effects or complications, particularly when taken in large amounts and over a long period of time. Some patients suffer more from "iatrogenic" or "treatment produced diseases" than from their arthritis.

The ARTHRITIS PROGRAM relies heavily on what may be called *natural methods.* The human body has a remarkable ability to repair itself and to cure diseases when assisted by the patient under medical supervision. For this reason climate, natural hot mineral water baths and exercise are given such an important place in the program.

Physical therapy is essential, especially at the beginning of treatment.

Diet, vitamins and minerals are used, to correct dietary deficiencies and therapeutically to build and restore the bone and joint damage of the arthritis patient. *Some medicines are used,* of course, *but not for long and not in larger amounts than absolutely necessary.* One of the best signs of improvement and recovery is the ability to decrease and finally discard the use of suppressive drugs.

Maximum improvement and recovery may be a matter of months, or years, but progress is seen in two or three weeks and continues as long as the program is followed.

A NOTE OF APPRECIATION

Credit should be given with highest praise and gratitude to our many hundreds of patients who were willing to try *something different,* natural foods, megavitamin therapy, herbs, vaccine, and the anti-protozoal drugs. They have made possible this compilation of therapeutic experiences which constitutes the medical wisdom on which this book is based.

RB, MD.

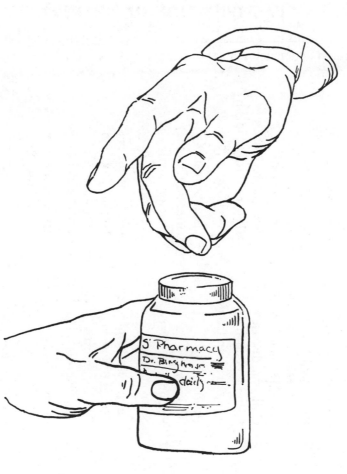

MEDICINES HELP - NATURE CURES

Table 1

A CLASSIFICATION OF ARTHRITIS

Arthritis may be associated with other systemic diseases and deficiencies. Two or more types may be present in a patient.

INFECTIOUS

Bacterial:
- Staphylococcal
- Gonococcal
- Tuberculosis
- Streptococcus
- Pneumococcus

Parasitic:
- Amoebic
- Malarial
- Treponemal

Viral:
- Hepatitis
- Mumps
- Rubella

Fungal:

Mycoplasmal:

INFLAMMATORY

- Rheumatoid
- Ankylosing spondylitis
- Juvenile rheumatoid
- Collagen disease
- Reiter's syndrome
- Sjogren's syndrome

- Psoriatic
- Polymyositis
- Rheumatic fever
- Scleroderma

- Lupus erythematosus
- Bechet's syndrome
- Polychrondritis
- Polyarteritis

- Polymyalgia

- Erthema nodosum

METABOLIC

- Osteoarthritis
- Traumatic
- Osteoporosis
- Aseptic necrosis
- Hyperparathyroidism
- Avascular necrosis

- Osteoporosis
- Allergic (Atopic)
- Calcium deficiency
- Vitamin D deficiency

- Osteochondrosis
- Hypothyroidism
- Hormonal deficiency
- Protein deficiency

- Hypertrophic osteo-arthropathy

- Gout

CHAPTER 1

THE MANY TYPES OF ARTHRITIS

"Arthritis is a large family of diseases.
ARTHRITIS IS USUALLY DEFINED **as a painful disease of the joints or related structures caused by inflammation or degeneration.** It is not a single disease but a large family of diseases—some closely related, some due to very different causes. When due to degeneration, rather than inflammation, the more correct word would be ARTHROSIS. The terms used in Europe and many other countries are RHEUMATISM and RHEUMATIC DISEASES. Whatever the name, they have one thing in common, abnormal tissue changes in the joints and related structures.

These diseases affect the mesenchymal tissues between the ectoderm (outside skin) and the entoderm (mucous membranes). During growth and development mesoderm forms the bones, joints (with their cartilage surfaces and linings, or synovia), muscles (with their tendons), ligaments (which hold joints together and form the body's "hinges"), and bursae (thin sacs of fluid over the joints at points of pressure and friction). These structures are enclosed in a network of fibrous connective tissue contained in the framework of all body parts. A main constituent of connective tissue is **collagen** (the "cement" substance of the body). Inflammatory and degenerative diseases that affect collagen are called the COLLAGEN DISEASES.[14]

SYMPTOMS

When the doctor says, "You probably have arthritis," the first question a patient usually asks is, "What kind of arthritis do I have?" His answer usually will be in general terms and rather evasive—and with good reason.

Most types of arthritis cannot be correctly diagnosed by the doctor on the first visit. Almost all kinds of arthritis are manifested by *joint pain, swelling, limitation of motion, local heat and inflammation* in one or more joints at the onset. The non-inflammatory conditions also show some pain, swelling and gradual joint enlargement but usually lack local heat, redness and signs of inflammation.

The first symptoms of arthritis often appear in the hands—with pain, soft swelling of the joints, increased warmth, redness, local inflammation and stiffness. In a person who has done a great deal of walking or standing the first signs may be in the feet or knees. Arthritis very frequently begins in joints that have been injured or weakened by overwork or some previous severe stress.

The doctor's final opinion will depend on the results of laboratory tests and x-ray reports which he will use to support his clinical diagnosis based on history and physical findings.

CLASSIFICATIONS OF ARTHRITIS

All types of arthritis are *acquired diseases.* No child is born with a rheumatic condition. Arthritis is not hereditary. Sometimes these conditions appear in several members of a family, or in several generations. But this is due to familial patterns of eating, dietary deficiencies, or exposure to similar toxic or infectious agents. **The joints you have when you are born should, with proper care and good health, last you for 100 years.**

Four situations, or any combination of these, can

bring on an attack of arthritis.
1. Infections caused by viruses, bacteria or protozoa.
2. Injuries, which damage the structure or the circulation of the bones or the joints.
3. Nutritional deficiencies, in protein, minerals or vitamins over a period of time.
4. Metabolic changes in the body. These may cause gout, osteoporosis, or the degenerative arthritis associated with arteriosclerosis, diabetes or nerve damage.

The two largest classes of joint diseases are those called rheumatoid arthritis and osteoarthritis. **RHEUMATOID ARTHRITIS** characteristically occurs in the knuckles (the metacarpal-phalangeal joints) and adjacent joints of the fingers (the proximal interphalangeal joints). These have large capsules containing joint fluid in proportion to their size and, in most people, are subject to more stress from use than any other joint of the body. This makes them ideal sites for the inflammatory involvement of the synovial membrane, the primary pathology in the rheumatoid arthritis joint.

OSTEOARTHRITIS, or **DEGENERATIVE ARTHRITIS** as it is frequently called, is usually indicated by gradual enlargement of the margins of the end (*distal* interphalangeal) joints of the fingers, which may occur without much pain or swelling. It may appear in the elderly along with similar changes in the spine or extremities, or prematurely in middle-age or younger as a result of injury or repeated minor stress or local trauma (as in the hands of typists, particularly before the introduction of electric typewriters). These diseases are discussed in more detail in the following chapter, but their differences should be kept in mind.

The general public seems to have the misconception that all arthritis is alike and can easily be relieved with the latest tablet or the television advertised rub-on lotion. There are more than 100 separate types.

GOUTY ARTHRITIS is a separate entity, due to a disorder of purine metabolism. It may occur first as small cystic sacs of fluid in the small joints at the ends of the fingers, or as often portrayed by the artist, as a swollen, red and painful great toe, elevated on a stool while the unhappy patient warns his visitors away. These tender and inflamed joints contain small and irritating crystals of uric acid. As the disease progresses these may become firm nodules, or "tophi", even found in the lobes of the ear.

DIAGNOSIS

The assistance of a physician is *very important* from the onset of the first symptoms of arthritis in order *to make an early clinical diagnosis.* Specific curative therapy is available for some bacteria-caused arthritis diseases such as staphylococcal or gonococcal arthritis. Arthritis due to tuberculosis or syphilis should have early chemotherapeutic treatment. Metabolic arthritis such as gout can be quickly corrected by dietary changes and some specific medications.

A good medical history will give the physician valuable clues to the type of arthritis the patient has. Did the symptoms follow an illness or disease at work, at home, or in recent travels? Does he have any chronic illnesses, allergies, or infections?

When the reaction of the body to the disease produces defense changes in the blood—as in rheumatoid arthritis and some of the rarer varieties of inflammatory arthritis—specific factors can be detected in the blood serum. Other *extensive laboratory tests required for an accurate diagnosis* must be repeated at regular intervals until the diagnosis and degree of severity of the disease is known. Some tests must be repeated as treatment progresses to determine any improvement or regression of the diseases. Ultimately, laboratory and x-ray examinations may make a definite diagnosis possible, which may take days, weeks, or even months.

However, a definite diagnosis of the *type* of arthritis may not be forthcoming. The laborabory tests may be "negative;" x-rays may show no significant changes; clinical signs and symptoms may not follow any definite clinical pattern. Then *the physician will treat a "clinical impression," or his best considered medical opinion, of the arthritis type.* He may refer the patient to a rheumatologist or a specialist in internal medicine for further examination and testing.

In a sample group of patients at the Desert Arthritis Medical Clinic in Desert Hot Springs, California, 47 had rheumatoid arthritis, 39 had osteoarthritis, 7 had gout, 14 had bursitis, 11 had fibrositis, and one had Reiter's syndrome. That totals 6 different diseases in a group of 119 patients; and the original diagnosis of 3 of these patients was incorrect and 70 of these patients had symptoms of two or more types of arthritis. This illustrates how *difficult it is for a physician to make a firm diagnosis* of the *type* of arthritis a patient has, particularly *early in the course of the disease.*[10]

MULTIPLE CAUSES OF ARTHRITIS

Diagnosis is further complicated by the fact that *a patient may have more than one type of arthritis;* or a disease that begins with one cause can later develop into a different type of arthritis. For example, an injury may cause an increase in synovial joint fluid, resulting in synovitis (joint swelling). A more severe injury can cause a *hemarthrosis,* a collection of blood and increased joint fluid; there may be damage to the cartilage and the adjacent bone, resulting in permanent joint damage. The patient then develops *post-traumatic arthritis,* or osteoarthritis due to the injury. Similarly, a patient may not recover completely from a joint infection or the infection may damage the blood supply to the joint, resulting in degenerative changes and osteoarthritis.

Records of the Desert Arthritis Medical Clinic indicate that *two out of three patients suffer from more than one kind of arthritis.* The resulting implications and consequences are just as important as finding another cause of arthritis.

The most common combinations found were: Osteoarthritis and osteoporosis, bursitis, Herberden's nodes, or gout; bursitis and degenerative disc disease, intervertebral disc degeneration, infectious arthritis, gout, or osteoarthritis. Less common but very frequent combinations were rheumatoid arthritis and bursitis, osteoporosis, infectious arthritis, degenerative disc disease, gout or osteoarthritis.

Many symptoms, laboratory tests, and x-rays must be considered in the diagnosis of two or more types of arthritis in the same patient. Even *three* types of arthritis (or three causes) have sometimes been found in the same patient. *It is ineffectual to treat only one type,* or only the most prominent symptoms *with a pain-relieving* or anti-inflammatory *drug without considering the whole patient*—his or her general health as well as physiological and chemical makeup. All possible causes of infectious, circulatory, or degenerative changes should be considered and treated. Only then can improvement and possible remission or "cure" be expected. *Both physician and patient must carefully search for more than one kind or cause of the arthritis* symptoms.

Consider the patient who has been under a doctor's care for months or years with *no improvement* and, even, a *downward progression* of his disease. The doctor discovers one type of arthritis and starts the conventional treatment. But the patient does not respond. Why? Because there are *two* types of arthritis. One type might be checked or controlled while the other advances and becomes worse.

When a patient has two types of arthritis, the treatment for one actually may be making the other type worse. For example, the various cortisone drugs give temporary relief of pain and swelling in active rheumatoid arthritis but cause and increase osteoporosis, another type of metabolic bone disease with the signs and symptoms of arthritis.[3]

Example. A patient has been treated for osteoarthritis with one of the usual pain-relieving or anti-inflammatory drugs. He has never had a blood chemistry panel (SMA). A very high uric acid level in his blood may indicate an active case of gout. On a program of exercise, physical therapy, a low purine diet, and small doses of an anti-gout drug he will be completely relieved of his pain within a week.

Example. A patient has multiple pains in his shoulders, hips, elbows, wrists, knees, and feet. X-rays show only small surface areas of joint sclerosis or occasional flecks of calcium over or near joint prominences. He has very early osteoarthritis, and physical findings show tenderness over these areas but no joint swelling or inflammation. His blood count shows an elevated number of white blood cells and polymorphic leukocytes, and he has a positive reaction to the vaccine test.

This patient has multiple bursitis and a focus of infection. A low-grade, chronic infection hides somewhere in his body; he has poor natural resistance and little or no immunity to these organisms. With arthritis vaccine injections, changes in diet and physical therapy he will be relieved of his chronic and disabling symptoms in a few weeks.

Example. Many women show enlargement of the joints of their hands—associated with increasingly poor posture and pain in the neck, upper back and shoulders. X-rays reveal both osteoarthritis and osteoporosis, resulting from years of low-calcium intake, lack of vitamin D, and a post-menopausal deficiency of ovarian hormone. They show immediate improvement during the initial three- to four-week course of examinations and treatments. Then they are started on a three- to four-month program which gradually eliminates pain in the spine, arrests joint deformities, and increases strength and function in their hands and other joints.

TWO OR MORE CAUSES?
TWO OR MORE DISEASES?

With *over 100 types and forms of arthritis,* the patient can find out if there is more than one type of disease only through complete clinical and laboratory evaluations. Medical history of the illness, the physical examination, x-rays of the affected bones and joints, chemical and serological examinations—all must be complete and extensive. These data then must be analyzed by a physician who not only treats the customary forms of arthritis but also is trained and qualified to discover the unusual types and complications.

POOR HEALTH AND ARTHRITIS

VARIOUS PATHOLOGICAL CONDITIONS contributing to arthritis concern the physician in diagnosis and treatment. Yet a large number of *seemingly unrelated factors may* also *affect the patient's health and* result in a predisposition to arthritis. When present, *any one of these factors may be the cause of arthritis.*

Good health is the basis for life itself; babies are born with it. But from then on it is a constant struggle against disease, dietary deficiency, the environment, stresses, accidents and injuries, and premature old age. *Improving the patient's general health is the number one treatment of arthritis. Arthritis can be prevented— even cured in some cases—by avoiding, removing, or diminishing conditions associated with its causes.*

Physicians can *treat* and *control* many diseases, but they care for a patient only *after* injury has occurred. All other aspects of good health are the responsibility of the individual and the public—parents for their children, government for its citizens, industries for their employees and customers, government and the drug industry for the protection of the public with safe foods, drugs, and nutritional supplements. The *arthritis patient should* be aware of all such influences and *use every method available to regain health, strength, and improved physical functions.*[23]

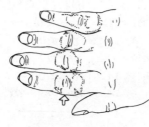
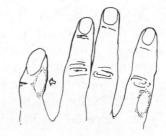

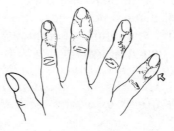

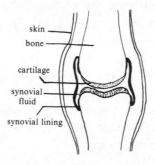
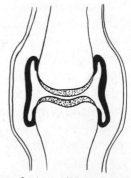

skin
bone
cartilage
synovial
fluid
synovial lining

1. Normal knee joint

2. Acute, inflamed

Rheumatoid Arthritis

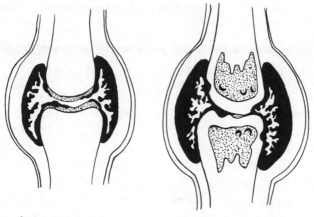

3. Severe arthritis   4. Chronic arthritis

Rheumatoid Arthritis

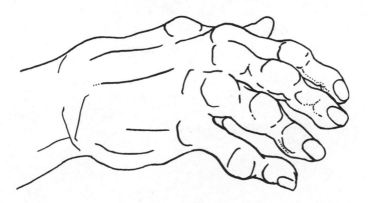

Osteoarthritis

Table 2

COMPARING RHEUMATOID ARTHRITIS AND OSTEOARTHRITIS

RHEUMATOID ARTHRITIS	OSTEOARTHRITIS
Inflammatory	Degenerative
Any age	Elderly patients
Unproven origin	Metabolic or traumatic
Acute onset	Gradual beginning
Moderate pain	Mild pain
Moderate swelling	Less swelling
Local heat and redness	Less heat and redness
Stiffness from swelling	Stiffness from joint damage
Loss of bone density (Osteoporosis)	Increased bone density (Osteosclerosis)
Origin probably from infection	Deficiency and circulatory in origin
Sedimentation Rate:	
Elevated	Normal
White blood count:	
Elevated	Normal
Hemoglobin:	
Lowered	Normal
Serological tests:	
Positive	Normal

Note: Not infrequently a patient may have both types of arthritis at the same time.

CHAPTER 2

RHEUMATOID ARTHRITIS AND OSTEOARTHRITIS

RHEUMATOID ARTHRITIS IN CHILDREN

Rheumatoid arthritis is the most serious crippling disease of childhood. It is more rare than poliomyelitis was during the epidemic years but is more devastating, as it shows a gradual progression in many cases. It is an active, recurrent, chronic disease which *may require medical care and treatment for a patient's entire life* since it often progresses and worsens with age.

No healthy, well-nourished child develops arthritis. In every case of juvenile rheumatoid arthritis (JRA) the child was weakened by injury, disease, stress, poor nutrition, or some pre-existing condition which lowered his resistance and presented a predisposing cause of the disease. Often the child will have more than one disease—arthritis plus some concomitant condition such as malnutrition, anemia, foci of infection, allergy, or gastrointestinal disturbances. These have to be treated along with the arthritis for the child to make a complete recovery.

There is more than one form of childhood arthritis. Some patients show joints that are hot, swollen, inflamed, enlarged, stiff, and painful; yet they may recover without damage. Others have joints which appear similar but suffer a loss of joint cartilage during the inflammatory stage, resulting in permanent stiffness, growth retardation, and atrophy. These may be two different manifestations of the same disease; or the infective agent may produce damage in one patient and no permanent joint changes in another.

PREDISPOSING CAUSES

The predisposing causes in older children and young adults may be similar: trauma, illness, injury, severe stress, or too rapid development. The most common factor is malnutrition, particularly a deficiency of vitamins C and D and calcium. *The child may have subclinical malnutrition.* Compared with healthy children of the same age there is always a difference. The rheumatoid child evidences delayed growth, poor physical development, loss of weight, less height for the same age, and subtle changes in the blood picture in laboratory examinations.

Early JRA patients are commonly found with anemia, high leukocyte counts, and slightly elevated sedimentation rates. They may also show synovitis of the joints, which may resolve completely with full recovery. The joints may be so highly inflamed that the joint fluid appears cloudy and purulent, as if full of pus, even when no organisms can be isolated. During surgery these joint linings will show a thickened, inflamed synovial membrane not much different from that of a bacterial infection.

TREATMENT OF JUVENILE ARTHRITIS

These patients must be treated with physical therapy, correction and protection of joint tendencies to deformities, and positive nutrition with therapeutic amounts of protein, natural carbohydrates, vitamins, and minerals. In the very early stages, when joints are hot, swollen, and tender, complete bedrest and gentle exercises to prevent stiffness are recommended. Antibiotics may be useful in the early stages, and arthritis vaccine may help the patient recover from the acute phase of the disease. Anti-protozoal drugs have been dramatic in the successful relief of several cases of JRA.

RHEUMATOID ARTHRITIS IN ADULTS

Between the ages of 30 and 50, *illnesses and repeated occupational injuries begin to play a role in the development of arthritis.* These include the common infections of early middle age in the teeth, tonsils, gastrointestinal tract, kidney, bladder, prostate, reproductive organs, and lungs. When organisms causing rheumatoid arthritis exist, they ride "piggyback" into the patient's body during or after some other infection. Stress, malnutrition, injury, surgery, and pregnancy can predispose to an attack of arthritis. Degenerative changes are not often symptomatic in this age group; but in considerably older patients their presence indicates that they were probably first evident, at least on x-ray, in the early 30's, 40's, and 50's.

Women in their 40's seem to have a predilection to rheumatoid arthritis in the hands, wrists, elbows, and shoulders because these joints are most used, overworked, or damaged by repeated heavy strains in household work. Their hands are especially susceptible and are more certain to develop degenerative arthritis.

RA IN ELDERLY PATIENTS

Rheumatoid arthritis is rare in elderly people, but some cases have developed in the 60's and 70's. These are often missed in the first examination because they are not expected in this age group. Rheumatoid arthritis appearing for the first time in a patient between 60 and 80 years old is usually considered to be an attack of painful osteoarthritis until all the physical and laboratory data confirming a rheumatoid arthritis diagnosis is at hand. During surgery some patients with clinical and x-ray findings of osteoarthritis were found to have active rheumatoid arthritis as well, with chronic synovitis, increased joint fluid, and inflammatory synovial joint linings; and yet these patients had no positive diagnostic tests for RA prior to operation.

THE CAUSES OF RHEUMATOID ARTHRITIS

Most clinical physicians (those who work with patients rather than only in laboratories) *believe there is an infectious agent in rheumatoid arthritis.* Onset of the disease is acute, with fever and elevated blood count, sedimentation rate, and white blood cell count. Joints are swollen, tender, hot, painful, and contain an excess of inflammatory joint fluid. Synovial fluid under the microscope shows inflammatory changes and an abnormal number of white blood cells (which increase in the presence of infection).

Laboratory tests in immunology may also indicate an infectious origin. Immune bodies found in the blood are similar to those which occur in the presence of infection. Varieties of specific immune bodies found in rheumatoid arthritis can often tell the doctor the type of rheumatoid arthritis, how active and severe it is, and how resistant it will be to treatment. Known arthritis-causing viruses occur in hepatitis, tick bites, and occasionally with systemic virus diseases such as rubella and the rare Lyme arthritis.[14]

One objection to the infectious origin of rheumatoid arthritis is the rarity of known cases of transmission from one person to another. But it can occur.

Example: Recently a young man with rheumatoid arthritis, who had been cared for continuously by his mother for 3 months, made a satisfactory recovery—

only to see his mother come down with the same type of rheumatoid arthritis disease.

Another objection is that conventional laboratory tests for viruses yield negative results. But this does not necessarily mean that a virus is not present. Very small viruses, called "picornaviruses" and "viroids," are so small they only show as particles in other cells.

Some agents used to treat rheumatoid arthritis may not work directly on the virus particles themselves but on the carriers of virus-causing agents—bacteria, protozoa, or other viruses.[20]

In 1969 a radiologist and an orthopedic surgeon found an agent in tissue drawn from rheumatoid arthritis patients which could be transmitted to mice and produce inflammatory changes. Since then, this infective agent has been found in the synovial joint tissues of patients with classical symptoms of rheumatoid arthritis. It is not found in chronic or advanced cases but seems to be present during the early and active stages when the disease is spreading from joint to joint.[39]

During 10 years of extensive laboratory tests, this infective agent was cultured in mice, rats, chickens, and fertile eggs. It was found to contain no protein or fat; it could not be identified as either a protozoa, bacteria, or virus. It survived temperatures (121° C. for 15 minutes) that would kill any known micro-organism. It was finally concluded that these infectious particles are composed of ribonucleic acid (RNA). They have no capsule or protective coatings and multiply when there is no inhibition or immunity present in the host body.

But the "questions" remain: *Do all rheumatoid arthritis patients harbor these infectious RNA particles?* How do they enter the body? How much are they affected by the body's immunity or inhibition? What will kill them or stop their growth?

CONFIRMING THE DIAGNOSIS

• Rheumatoid arthritis is suspected when x-rays reveal a loss of calcium and cartilage joint space near the ends of the bones or in the joints. Elevation of the sedimentation rate or positive arthritis serology tests are also helpful in this diagnosis. Other findings include:

> • An increased number of white blood cells may indicate chronic inflammation or infection.

> • An increase in the lymphocytes compared with the polymorphonuclear cells may lead to a diagnosis of a chronic virus infection.

> • An increase in the monocytes may suggest a granulomatous infection.

> • A "shift to the left", or polymorphonuclear predominance, may lead to the discovery of a bacterial infection.

> • A strong antistreptolysin titer (ASOT) may result in finding a chronic streptococcus infection in the body.

> • An increase in the number of eosinophils in the blood may indicate the presence of an allergy, or a gastrointestinal infection— particularly of the protozoa recently linked with some types of rheumatoid arthritis.

OSTEOARTHRITIS

The first symptoms of osteoarthritis are often seen in the hands and feet. *Gradual enlargement of the joints, with increased stiffness, are the presenting symptoms* often accompanied by mild, chronic pain and swelling that moves from joint to joint. The feet are painful when standing or walking; the toes gradually become deformed. The patient notices a weakness in the grasp of his hands and is unable to walk any long distance. X-rays show a loss of cartilage and narrowing of the joint spaces in the hands and feet. *Physical examination shows impaired circulation. The joints,* may be soft, tender, and slightly warmer than normal. These patients are more susceptible to cold and fatigue.

The hands and feet may suffer from poor circulation. Hardening of the arteries affects not only the heart or brain but also impairs circulation to the joints in the hands and feet. The cartilage and joint capsules receive less blood, oxygen, and nourishment; a gradual deterioration of the joint begins.

Such *patients are often found to be on a diet deficient in calcium and vitamins E and D.* Their joints have become soft, tender, and painful to the pressures of grasping or walking because the bone is soft and the cartilage is undergoing gradual degeneration. Repeated stress or strain on these joints causes them to spread, becoming stiff and enlarged, in the same way that a wooden stake spreads at the top when hit with a hammer.

MINERAL DEFICIENCIES

The most common dietary deficiency is calcium. Women particularly stop drinking milk because it is "too fattening," "causes mucus," or they just "don't like it." As a result they suffer from soft bones, muscle cramps, and enlarged, painful joints. When this lack of calcium is associated with lack of vitamin D and ovarian hormone, the progress of osteoarthritis and osteoporosis is even greater.[9]

FAMILIAL ARTHRITIS

Enlargement of the end joints of the fingers (called Heberden's nodes) in some patients (usually women) seems to run in patterns from grandmother to mother to daughter. This is the only type of arthritis which might be considered "hereditary." But a study of these patients reveals that most have a similar pattern of diet from one generation to another: Too much bread and spaghetti; not enough calcium, fish, liver, or food oil. Regardless of heredity, the pain and enlargement of Heberden's nodes can be greatly decreased by proper nutritional management and improved bone and joint circulation.

ARTHRITIS IN ELDERLY PATIENTS

Degenerative arthritis, or osteoarthritis, is the most common diagnosis in older patients and is one of the earliest signs of physical degeneration, or "old age." It may be predisposed by a single trauma or by repeated moderate trauma such as occupational injury. It may follow debilitating illness. *It is certainly related to a dietary deficiency, particularly of calcium and vitamin D, and is* often associated with other degenerative conditions of the soft tissues (such as intervertebral disc degeneration in the cervical, thoracic, and lumbar spine or bursitis in the shoulders, elbows, wrists, hips, knees, and feet). It is not unusual for arthritis to develop in middle-aged patients who have had since childhood chronic deformities of the bones and joints such as knock knees, bow legs, tibial torsion, and dysplasia of the hips.[3]

WEARING SHOES

Improper footwear—particularly those designed for style rather than comfort—frequently contribute to the development of degenerative changes in the joints and osteoarthritis of the feet.

Traumatic arthritis (osteoarthritis that develops in damaged joints) may be caused by single joint injuries or repeated joint strains in excess of what the body was made to stand. It may follow fractures or dislocations in areas of the bone that have suffered damage to the circulation of the joint surfaces; or it may develop more gradually from repeated stress associated with nutritional deprivation during growth and development.

In children this may be seen as osteochondritis of the spine, a pathological condition of development such as slipped epephysis of the hip or Perthe's disease.

Traumatic arthritis is frequently seen with poorly developed bone—the tissues show a lack of bone calcium, delayed bone growth and development, and inadequate repair after injury or deformity (whether from natural or surgical means).

OSTEOPOROSIS

The *elderly often show advanced degrees of osteoporosis,* a condition of calcium and protein deficiency affecting the collagen tissues (bone, cartilage, ligaments, tendons, muscle fascia sheaths, and connective tissues of the skin). The loss of cartilage in involved joints produces narrowing of the joint space and proportionate degrees of disability. Since *cartilage is not* usually *seen in x-rays, destruction is considered present when the joint space is narrowed.* When the space becomes completely obliterated, bone rubs on bone and pain with increasing joint stiffness follows. Ligaments and joints may loosen or relax, producing instability. At this stage, surgical reconstruction of the joints is usually necessary to restore stability and function, relieve the pain of motion, and permit better locomotion.[10]

Conservative core of patients with osteoporosis is a prolonged treatment but may be successful. It includes a special diet, calcium—usually from milk, phosphorus from vegetables and vitamin D from food supplements, vitamin C to build collagen, and for post-menopausal women hormone supplements may be indicated.

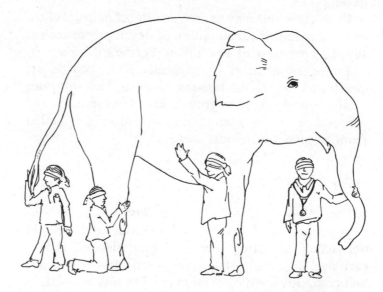

THE RHEUMATOID ELEPHANT
AND THE BLINDFOLDED DOCTORS
— IS THE CAUSE INFECTION?
ALLERGIC?, IMMUNE DEFICIENCY?,
HEREDITARY?, ETC.?

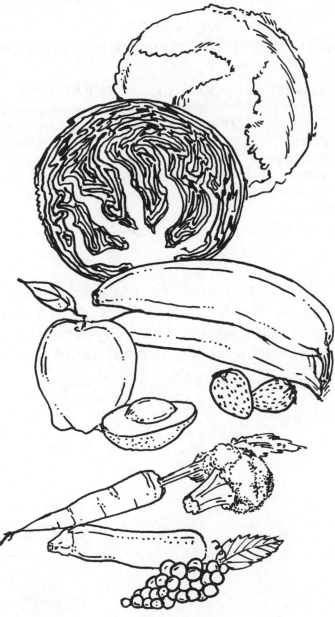

NATURAL FOODS ARE BEST

Table 3

NUTRITIONAL DEFICIENCIES IN ARTHRITIS

DEFICIENCY	RESULT	TREATMENT
Calcium	Osteoporosis	Milk and dairy foods
Protein	"	Meat, eggs, grains
Phosphates	"	Vegetables
Vitamin C	Weak bone	Fruit and juices
Trace minerals	"	Vegetables
Flouride	"	Water
Vitamin D	"	Fish liver oils

Deficiencies in other vitamins and minerals may be factors in the onset of arthritis. These can be prevented by a multiple vitamin-mineral supplement taken daily.

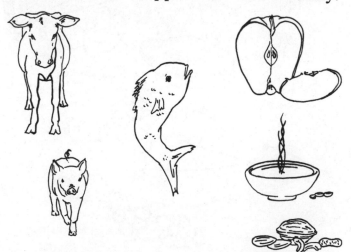

FRESH FOODS ARE BEST

CHAPTER 3

NUTRITIONAL DEFICIENCY

There is no medical proof that arthritis is hereditary. *Some families,* living in the same environment from generation to generation, *develop nutritional deficiencies* because of national or racial food patterns. These *deficiencies can predispose* to arthritis more in some families than others.

It was once believed that American Indians had a hereditary predisposition to arthritis. So in 1939 Dr. Weston Price visited isolated Indian tribes of the Yukon Territory. "Careful inquiry regarding the presence of arthritis was made in the more isolated groups. We neither saw nor heard of a case." But at the point of contact with white men—especially along the railroad *where the Indians had adopted white man's food—many cases of arthritis were found,* including bedridden cripples in 10 out of 20 Indian families. He found many of the younger generation crippled with arthritis.

Price proved that rheumatic fever, rheumatism, arthritis, and osteoporosis were rare or nonexistent in isolated peoples of the world—especially in Switzerland, Ireland, Canada, Melanesia, Polynesia, Africa, Australia, New Zealand, and Peru. Modern races in contact with civilized foods showed an increase in all of the bone and joint diseases, even in the same generation.

Odum visited these same areas 20 years later and reported *an increase in degenerative diseases among primitive peoples who were changing to "civilized" foods.*

The history of man on earth is too short to indicate any significant hereditary changes due to diet. Like our ancestors, *our bodies are designed to maintain health with pure water, natural fruits and vegetables,* and a certain amount of cooked foods such as vegetables, meat, fish, and eggs. Natural dairy products have always had an important role in the diet of man.

But when these foods are overcooked, processed, preserved, canned, bottled, pasteurized, dehydrated, or chemically preserved with additives they are degraded in various ways. Some of the natural vitamins and digestible food factors are lost. Additives interfere with digestion, absorption, and nutrition.[46]

THE FIRST RULE FOR GOOD HEALTH

Consequently, *foods should be taken from natural sources and served in their natural states as much as possible.*[11]

There is ample clinical evidence supporting the relationship of poor nutrition and the onset of arthritis.

Wyatt claims *it is possible to benefit 9 out of 10 chronic arthritis patients through a program of applied nutrition, but* he maintains *there is no such thing as an arthritis diet that can be adopted by every patient.* He believed that adequate nutritional therapy required investigating the patient's individual deficiencies, imbalances of dietary intake, and ability to utilize food items—then formulating a personal nutritional program containing the essential nutrients.[61]

Pearson investigated the relationship of rheumatic fever, one of the family of rheumatoid diseases, to nutritional deficiencies. In a dietary analysis of 93 rheumatic fever patients he found only 8 with a sufficient protein intake, only 4 with the normal amounts of calcium and trace minerals, and only one with the normal intake of vitamin C. Vitamin B-complex and D factors were low or nearly absent in many of these patients. On the other hand, these *children and young adults showed an abnormally high intake of refined sugars and carbohydrates.*[45]

PROTEIN DEFICIENCY VS EXCESS CARBOHYDRATES

The steady increase in arthritis in civilized countries parallels the gradual decrease in high protein foods (milk, meat, fish, poultry, nuts and whole grains) and the resulting increase in consumption of refined carbohydrates (white flour, white sugar, and processed and convenience foods). *Most arthritics seem to have an increased desire or craving for the very foods which contribute most to the worsening of their condition— sweets and starches.*[61]

LOW CALORIE DIETS

The total caloric intake may not be high—in fact, many patients are on weight-reducing diets—yet their carbohydrate intake is often abnormally high, with an excess of acid-producing foods. Since most vitamins and minerals are found in protein foods, most arthritic patients are also deficient in these important factors for the health and preservation of muscles and joints.

FAT CONSUMPTION

The fat intake of most patients is nearly normal or only slightly elevated, even in overweight patients, indicating that their excess weight is from a high carbohydrate intake rather than too much fat in the diet. *Some fat patients have a high intake of cottonseed oil, which produces a type of fat on the lower half of the body (abdomen, buttocks, thighs, and legs) which is very difficult to remove even with dieting and exercise.* It is poorly metabolized in the body and may even obstruct the smaller arteries which supply blood to the joints. Since cottonseed oil shortenings are cheaper than other food oils, they are almost invariably found in commercial bakery goods, which many arthritis patients consume in abnormal amounts.

CHILDREN'S DIETS

The *diets of juvenile arthritis patients are usually excessively high in carbohydrates:* refined sugar in the form of breads, desserts, candy, soft drinks, and "junk" foods.

DIETS OF ELDERLY PATIENTS

The *diets of older patients are more commonly low in protein and calcium from a lack of milk and dairy products.* These patients invariably have osteoarthritis or osteoporosis, or both. Protein and calcium are well supplied by milk, buttermilk, yogurt, cottage cheese, butter and cheese, and are essential "arthritis protective foods".

VITAMIN DEFICIENCIES

Most patients on the "average American diet" (supposedly the "world's best" and not requiring additional vitamins or food supplements) *receive only about 5% of their normal daily requirement of vitamin D.* Since it is essential for bone metabolism and has been found to act as a steroid hormone, any vitamin D deficiency results in joint damage and lack of bone replacement and repair.

Vitamins B and C are below normal in most arthritis patients, and invariably low in cases of rheumatoid arthritis. Chronic low intake of these vitamins predisposes to lowered resistance against disease, particularly those of viral origin which long have been suspected in the cause of rheumatoid disease. They are water soluble and not stored in the body, so they must be obtained in fresh fruits and vegetables, nuts, and grains.

Depletion of the B-complex and C vitamins occurs in stress and exhaustion, after surgical operations, illnesses, and injuries. A deficiency of only a short time can make a patient's joints more susceptible to the onset of acute arthritis.

Unexpected deficiencies which produce a sort of "metabolic poor health" do not necessarily cause arthritis but certainly decrease the chances of recovery. *Iron deficiency is frequent, especially in female patients,* and is almost always associated with proportionally low levels of the essential trace minerals—phosphorus, magnesium, iodine, copper, chromium, cobalt, manganese, molybdenum, selenium, and zinc. Although the individual need for some of these factors cannot be measured, a diet low in iron is poor in foods which come from the soil.

In order to adequately determine a patient's nutritional deficiencies and take steps to correct them, laboratory analysis is essential. Physical and x-ray examinations usually reveal the nature and extent of his disease; but laboratory tests will show whether it is acute or chronic, arrested or spreading, improving or becoming worse. *The type and degree of dietary deficiency in the patient's body can be determined by means of a detailed "dietary analysis", and a "hair analysis for trace minerals".*[49]

CALCIUM DEFICIENCY

One of the chief causes of arthritis in many patients is calcium deficiency—whether it is a simple lack of nutritional calcium in the diet or a disturbance in the body's metabolism of calcium.

An adequate calcium intake is absolutely necessary, regardless of age. Milk is the best natural food source. *The physical growth and development of infants nursed by their mothers is always superior—* particularly the skeletal and bone structure—to that of children raised on the bottle, no matter what the formula content. (The only possible exceptions are infants raised on certified raw milk.) They also have better bone and joint development than children raised on pasteurized milk, particularly in the width of their shoulders and pelvis and the development of their jaw structures; they have less crowding of the teeth and more symmetrical development of the facial bones.

The most beautiful and healthy children are those raised on raw milk on the farm, in the Scandinavian countries, or in areas such as Southern California where certified raw milk is widely available.

Milk is a great growth stimulus because it contains a growth hormone intended to change a calf into a heifer in a year. Removing the cream reduces some of these useful hormone and vitamin factors; but pasteurized, low fat, skim, and buttermilk are still excellent sources of calcium. For those who cannot take milk, enzyme tablets can help in the digestion of lactose; and other milk products such as cottage cheese, yogurt, keifer, and natural cheese may be substituted. Calcium tablets prepared from organic sources such as bone meal or oyster shells are superior to the purely chemical inorganic mineral compounds found in many commercially-prepared supplements.

Absorption of calcium in the gastrointestinal system depends partly on the presence of hydrochloric acid in the stomach. Those who take excessive amounts of alkali or antacids for indigestion, or large amounts of buffered aspirin for pain, or patients with atrophy of the gastrointestinal lining may be deficient in hydrochloric acid. Dilute hydrochloric acid may be sipped through a straw (so it will not damage teeth) after meals, or glutamic acid tablets may be taken. Honey and vinegar as a folk remedy for arthritis may be successful because it stimulates the formation of hydrochloric acid in the stomach; and the acid in the vinegar aids in calcium absorption.

Chocolate interferes with the absorption and digestion of calcium and should not be eaten regularly or frequently, especially by children and elderly persons.[57]

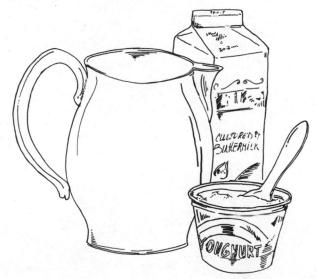

DAIRY PRODUCTS — THE BEST SOURCE OF CALCIUM

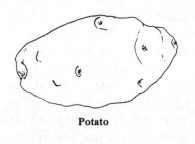

Potato

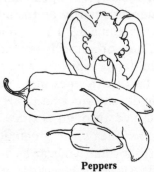

Peppers

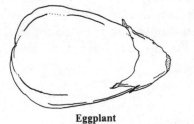

Eggplant

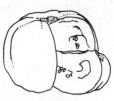

Tomato

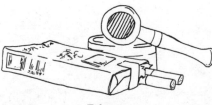

Tobacco

PLANTS HIGH IN SOLANINES

NO SOLANINE DIET

Arthritis is one of the diseases which is aggravated by the nightshade plants which are (*white potato, tomato, eggplant, red pepper* and *tobacco*). The "no nightshades" diet advocated by Dr. Childers demands *absolute avoidance* of these solanine-containing plants and their products. In 50% of arthritis patients even small amounts of the nightshades will keep the problem active, with pain and other symptoms being delayed until 2-4 days later. Flare-ups are nearly always due to taking in bits of nightshades inadvertently

Dr. Childers claims that everyone who adheres rigidly to this diet will get good results. *Prevention* magazine has data from over 900 cooperators on the diet, 87% showing favorable results.

In addition to solanines, all forms of tobacco carry toxic nicotine substances into the blood and tissues, which are especially damaging to muscle and nerve metabolism.

Table 4

FOUR FOODS AND ONE PLANT WHICH MAY CAUSE ARTHRITIS

THE "NIGHTSHADE" PLANTS AND VEGETABLES

Food allergies are a major problem in fifty per cent of patients with arthritis, compared with only five percent of allergy to foods in otherwise healthy persons.

The *solanine* containing foods have been found toxic to many arthritis patients. These are:

White potatoes	*Solanum tuberosum*
Eggplant	*Solanum melongena*
Tomatoes	*Lycopersicum esculentum*
Red peppers	*Capsicum ssp.*

Other nightshade plants *(Solanaceae)* are ground cherries and *tobacco* (which contains both nicotine and solanine). Common symptoms are pain and joint stiffness.

While recovering from an attack of arthritis it is very strongly recommended that patients eliminate these four foods from their diets and abstain from smoking tobacco.

CHAPTER 4

ALLERGY AND THE NIGHTSHADES

CLINICAL EVIDENCE indicates that ALLERGY is the major cause of arthritis in some patients. Many rheumatologists subscribe to the theory that patients with rheumatoid arthritis have become allergic to themselves. This is the reason that RA is often called auto-immune disease. Research in immunology has isolated many blood factors which seem to support this hypothesis. However the reaction of the human body to viruses, microplasms and protozoa may also be initiating these responses. For this reason patients must choose for themselves among many treatments for arthritis. Until further discoveries and proof establish the cause of inflammatory arthritis, no treatment which has been shown to help some patients should be condemned by the medical profession. Because it takes hundreds of thousands of dollars, even millions in the case of new drugs, to prove the worth of a treatment by animal experiments and double blind, random selection, scientific, clinical trials—no natural or biological remedy for arthritis should be rejected for lack of statistical proof of its effectiveness. Each treatment should be judged on its risk vs. benefit to patients.

FOOD ALLERGY is a primary cause of arthritis in many patients with several forms of arthritis. It is an aggravating factor in other rheumatoid diseases. Processed foods seem to be more at fault in this regard than natural foods—whose active enzymes help digest food components. Elimination diets will disclose the offending foods by a preliminary period of fasting, (we recommend three days) then introducing one food at a

time and noting the appearance of arthritis or any
other adverse reactions. CYTOTOXIC TESTING for
food allergies is also available in some medical centers,
determining the sensitivities to a great variety of foods
and other allergens by examining a specimen of the
patient's blood. This test is not yet accepted by most
rheumatologists but has proved invaluable in some
cases.

Example. A typical 58-year-old male patient was found
allergic to corn, wheat, rice, cane sugar, milk, beef, and
gas combustion products in his home. Avoiding these
foods and changing his heating system dramatically
corrected his arthritis. Prior to this treatment he had
undergone conventional therapy for synovitis and was
walking on crutches due to a painful, swollen knee. He
has remained free of arthritis for the past 7 years,
playing golf and tennis and running daily.[49]

Ample evidence in the medical literature implicates
food allergy as one cause of rheumatoid arthritis,
although this has been largely ignored except for a
handful of pioneering allergists. Turnbull treated 127
cases by eliminating skin test positive foods, with 59%
success in relieving all symptoms.[57] Zeller obtained
four well documented cures and observed striking
improvement of joint conditions that originally
appeared irreversible.[65] One patient was sensitive only
to beef; another reacted to lettuce, potatoes, and string
beans. Zussman[66] obtained three similar cures but was
hesitant to admit to it, stating simply that his patients
had "food sensitivity simulating rheumatoid
arthritis."[66] Rowe presented 25 successful treatments
and detailed histories in his food allergy textbook.[49] A
comprehensive medical review by Millman strongly
implicated allergy in rheumatoid arthritis. Dong claims
to have cured "thousands" of arthritics, directly and

through his popular books, with a fixed, low-allergen diet avoiding meat, milk, fruit, egg yolk, chocolate, and hot spices.[40]

Randolph summarized his 25-year experience with over 200 rheumatoid arthritis cases, *many cases are complicated by sensitivity to environmental chemicals,* by observing that *rheumatoid arthritics respond to allergy treatment "with but rare exceptions."*[47] Indeed, most of the clinical evidence cited demonstrates a clear cause-and effect relationship between foods eaten and arthritic pain. In over 232 cases from four independent investigators the following observations were made.

● *Acute arthritic symptoms disappeared following a restricted (or fasting) diet for 5 to 7 days.*
● Symptoms recurred when certain foods were individually restored to the diet.
● Symptoms disappeared again when each such food was withdrawn.
● Most patients experienced several cycles of symptom production and remission in response to foods.
● No regression was observed when patients continued with normal diets from which only the offending foods were eliminated (except when a patient injudiciously ate allergenic food).

The systemic symptoms of rheumatoid arthritis (fatigue, weakness, and fever) are also symptomatic of allergic toxemia. The typical remissions and exacerbations, including frequent remission in pregnancy, are also observed in bronchial asthma, a lung allergy. Acute isolated arthritis attacks may have the same duration as isolated food allergy attacks (usually 3 to 7 days). *Food allergy symptoms typically exacerbate during the night or early morning, perhaps accounting for arthritic morning stiffness.*

The rheumatoid blood factor, an antibody which builds up as the disease progresses, may be a response to sustained allergenic stimulus.[14] Typical joint pathology involves unmistakable immunological phenomena. The arthritis which accompanies many infectious diseases may show typical allergy symptoms.

Some people may be allergic only to processed foods, such as canned fruit and fruit juices, *while they are able to eat fresh foods with no reaction.* This suggests an allergy to the preservative or additive rather than the food itself. *Some patients supposedly allergic to milk* are really sensitive to processed milk and the changes produced by pasteurization and homogenization; they *may in fact, be able to drink raw milk with no difficulty.* If sensitive to raw cow's milk they can sometimes substitue goat's milk. Whole grains such as oatmeal and granola are better tolerated than processed cereals or bread.[65]

Many people are allergic to corn in any form: canned or fresh corn, popcorn, and corn sugar such as found in candies, steak sauce, and artificial dairy creamers.

SOLANINE ALLERGIES

The solanine-containing *"nightshade"* foods are highly toxic to many arthritis patients, especially when consumed over a period of months or years. *Solanines may be the only cause of arthritis in some patients;* in *others,* a secondary cause that interferes with their recovery. The *solanine foods include white potatoes, tomatoes, eggplant, all types of peppers* (except black pepper), *and tobacco in any form.*

THE NIGHTSHADE PLANTS

The large nightshade family of plants (Solanaceae)

native to tropical America is one of the leading sources of foods, drugs, and ornamental plants. Important food plants include the potato, eggplant, ground cherries, red peppers, and tomato. Drugs include nicotine (from *Nicotiana*), belladonna and atropine (from *Atropa*), henbane (from *Hyoscyamus*), and stramonium (from *Datura*).

Certain of these plants, however, contain *toxic chemicals (solanines) that cause illness, even death, in humans and animals when ingested in quantities above the "safe level,"* including the highly toxic black and deadly nightshades.

The origin of the English term "nightshades" may be their "evil and loving nature of the night." According to Childers and Russo,[26] "The Romans in the old days were said to prepare potions of the deadly nightshades and offer them to their enemies . . . 'the shade came down for a long night.' "

In a special scientific study on the relation of nightshades to arthritis and health, Childers and Russo found *toxic amounts of dangerous solanines in the four common nightshade food plants*—white potatoes, eggplant, tomatoes, and garden peppers—and in tobacco. Completely eliminating these foods from the diet brought relief and even recovery to some 3,000 arthritis patients.

THE NUTRITIONAL APPROACH

The medical profession has long been resistant to the nutritional treatment of arthritis and other degenerative diseases. Most medical college programs do not include sufficient training in plant, animal, and human nutrition. *Teaching and research is centered mainly in developing new drugs, new technology,* surgery, psychiatry, and other approaches to *treat the symptoms of disease rather than to seek nutritional causes.* But these new discoveries may produce a rapid change in the thinking and practice of many doctors.

No arthritis patient can be considered completely and thoroughly treated without a thorough trial of the "no-nightshades" diet.

Even though the nightshade foods probably amount to less than 10% of the population's diet, they play such a large role in American life and habits that it is difficult to reduce or eliminate them, even with arthritis patients. Yet studies in progress indicate that *over 50% of arthritis patients suffer some toxic effects from nightshades in the cause or aggravation of their disease.*

Small amounts of these foods are probably toxic only over many years, which may explain why some forms of arthritis, such as hypertropic osteoarthritis, appear more often in the later years of life. But in areas of the world where the nightshade plants are not used as food, this form of the disease is much less prevalent than in the Western World. The no-nightshades diet is generally known in South Africa and Rhodesia, where natives from the north who came to the Cape Town area with little or no arthritis developed typical arthritic symptoms after a few months on local menus.

SYMPTOMS OF SOLANINE TOXICITY

Kingsbury found that the symptoms and lesions caused by the various types of nightshade plants were quite similar, even though their chemical composition is somewhat different. The *plants contain a saponic-like* glycoalkaloid, an irritant *causing red blood cell destruction, and a toxic steroid alkamine,* which is absorbed through the intestine and *responsible for nervous symptoms in both animals and man.*[35]

When these chemicals are absorbed into the body in sufficient quantity, they cause anorexia (loss of appetite), nausea, dizziness, abdominal pain, vomiting, constipation or diarrhea (sometimes with blood), anemia, weakness, and accumulation of fluid in the abdomen. Inflammation can occur in the gastrointestinal tract with ulceration, hemorrhage, and diverticulitis. Cases of acute poisoning are rare but can contribute to the death of the weak or elderly. Nervous effects from these toxic substances include apathy, drowsiness, salivation, difficulty in breathing, trembling, progressive weakness to the extent of paralysis, prostration, and eventually unconsciousness. Solanine poisoning is not always fatal; but death, when it occurs, is probably from paralysis of the heart.

The *most common efects of chronic or low-level solanine poisoning is pain and stiffness. It can occur in the back of many joints and their related muscles and* tendons, with joint swelling and skin rash. Solanine is an inhibitor of cholinesterase, an enzyme that provides agility of muscle movements. Lack of this enzyme can cause stiffness and slow muscle movement. The joint pain swelling, and stiffness frequently are associated with gastrointestinal symptoms and nerve problems. Patients who have recovered after eliminating nightshades from their diet had been previously diagnosed as "chronic arthritis," "multiple arthritis," "osteoarthritis," and even "rheumatoid arthritis."

POTATO *SOLANUM TUBEROSUM*

The white potato is the most common of the nightshade foods. It originates from Peru and has been used as human food for about 400 years. Glycolkaloid and solanine is present throughout the potato, with the most concentration in the peel. Farmers have found that cattle and horses eating potato vines frequently become ill, develop nervous symptoms and paralysis, and may even die. These toxic reactions are known to growers, who attempt to keep the solanine content below 20mg/100gm of fresh potatoes, which is thought to be safe for human consumption.

The white potato may give a tranquilizing effect within an hour after eating; then aches and pains set in within the next day or so.

Besides being eaten whole as a staple in the diet of many people, potatoes are also processed into many prepared foods. Potato products and potato starch (for body) are found in baby foods, inexpensive yogurts, gravies, and sauces.

It is interesting to note that, when first introduced into Europe by 16th century Spanish explorers, potatoes were at first shunned as food because many people thought they were poisonous!

TOMATO *LYCOPERSICUM ESCULENTUM*

As an excellent source of vitamins A and C, the tomato has become an important food in the civilized world; its use as a food has increased markedly in the United States in this century. However, it was believed to be poisonous throughout Europe except for Italy, where it has been used as a dietary staple.

Besides its use as a fresh food, tomatoes are found in a wide variety of processed foods for flavoring such as sauces, baby foods, and other prepared foods.

Tomato vines are poisonous to livestock; *just handling tomatoes or their vines will cause sore, inflamed hands in some people.* One woman claims that nursing her baby after eating tomato products will cause it to cry all day.

RED PEPPER *CAPSICUM SPP.*

Three main varieties of red peppers contain solanines: the sweet, or bell pepper; paprika, or pimiento; and chili, or cayenne pepper. Not included are the black and white peppers of Piperaceae family which are commonly used as table seasonings.

Chili peppers often used in Mexican-style food contain solanines that *can irritate the gastrointestinal tract, cause skin rash, and may contribute to* the *development of arthritis.* Use of paprika may immediately produce tingling in the chest area, then in the legs and arms; and later, pain may settle in a different joint at different times. Pinkish, colored cheeses often contain paprika.

Other *products that often contain red pepper* in various forms *are herb teas, cough lozenges, pain ointments, gravies and sauces* (such as Tobasco and *barbeque sauces*), *and certain brands of vitamin C tablets which contain peel oil.*

EGGPLANT SOLANUM MELONGENA

Less popular, the eggplant has been used for food only in the present century. It was thought to cause insanity in the Mediterranean area if eaten daily for as long as a month.

TOBACCO *NICOTIANA TABACUM*

The harmful effects of nicotine in tobacco are well known; but few are aware of its toxic solanine content.[35]

Smoking could be called a "double whammy" injuring arthritis patients two ways.

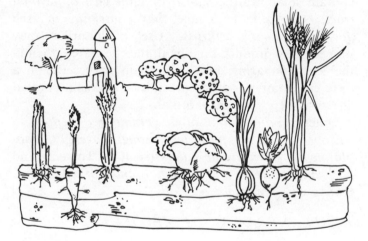

FARM FRESH IS BEST

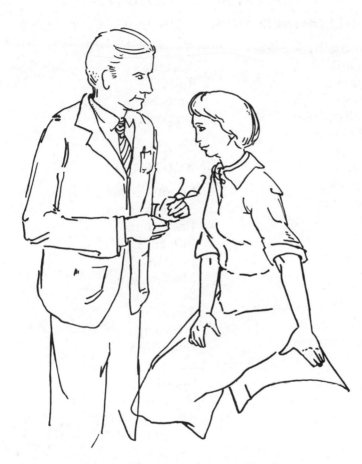

YOUR PHYSICIAN SHOULD SEARCH
FOR ANY FOCI OF INFECTION

Table 5

INFECTIONS IN ARTHRITIS

FOCI OF INFECTIONS

CHRONIC INFECTIONS

Teeth
tonsils
sinuses
lungs
gall bladder
intestines
colon
kidney
bladder
prostate
uterus
boils
abscesses
acne
wounds
surgical operations
osteomyelitis
joint infections
and infectious diseases.

Viruses
bacteria
fungi
amoebae
mycoplasmas.

ACUTE INFECTIONS

Streptococcus
Staphlococcus
Pneumonia
Influenza
Measles
Mumps
Scarlet Fever
Tonsillitis
Septicemia
Gonorrhea
Syphilis
Colitis
Hepatitis
Rheumatic Fever
and fevers of "unknown
     origin".

CHAPTER 5

INFECTION

Though less common than years ago, infections are still important contributing causes, or even the sole cause, of arthritis symptoms or disease in many patients.

Potential infections are always around us in viruses, bacteria, and protozoa, which can combine with each other to act against us. Our only protections against infection is good health, our immune system, and nutrition—especially adequate vitamin and mineral intake.

Everyone is born with a degree of natural immunity, transmitted to the newborn baby from the bloodstream of its mother. It is created by the action of the reticuloendothelial cells just under the surface of the skin and by the formation of infection-fighting white blood cells in the bone marrow. *After exposure to minimal amounts of infectious agents, the body responds by developing further immunity. Medically it is produced by vaccines, antigens*, and substances containing antibodies such as immune globulin.

A lowered immunity may result in arthritis of infectious origin.

FOCI OF INFECTION

Chronic dental infection, retained roots, and infected gums should be investigated and treated by a dentist. Dental x-rays may uncover dead or unextracted roots, unsuspected abscesses, osteoporosis, or pyorrhea. Chronic infection of the paranasal sinuses and infected lymphoid tissues in the throat and tonsils are also accessible to medical examination and treatment. A routine chest x-ray occasionally shows chronic bronchitis, rheumatoid disease of the lungs, bronchiectasis, and, in California, unsuspected cases of "valley fever." Tuberculosis is rare but still very present, particularly in metropolitan areas.

Infections in the liver, gallbladder, gastrointestinal systems, appendix, kidneys, bladder, prostate, or uterus may be insidious and the source of inflammatory arthritis.

LABORATORY FINDINGS

An increase in white blood count, elevated sedimentation rate, or infection as shown by urinalysis may be the first clues. *An increase in eosinophils* in the white blood count, either in percentage or total numbers, *may signify intestinal infection* with protozoa, *amenable to treatment with the anti-protozoal drugs in rheumatoid* arthritis patients.

TREATMENT

Some of the new, alternative treatments—such as use of the "rediscovered" arthritis vaccines—cannot be proven effective by statistical analysis, animal research, or laboratory controls. But clinical evidence demonstrated by improvement in hundreds of arthritis patients is impressive.

The clinical effects of large doses of vitamin C in viral infections and in arthritis have been confirmed in hundreds of patients since the early 1950's, when Dr. Fred Klenner found vitamin C effective in the treatment of poliomyelitis. *Therapeutic amounts of vitamin C are recommended in the treatment of all forms of arthritis,* and some day the evidence may prove that it *prevents*[30] some types of arthritis as well as some types of cancer.

PROTOZOA

Our environment contains free-living amoeba on the surface soil and in fresh water. They form cysts which float in the air and are continually inhaled. They are found in the nasopharynx, and their trophozoites are present in human and animal feces. Amoebae (*Naegleria* spp.) are found in healthy human tissue, and exist in large numbers in human cancer tissue, and in tissue taken from cases of rheumatoid disease. The presence of these amoebae in the body represents the source of constant antigenic stimulation believed responsible for rheumatoid disease as well as the development of myelomatosis and lymphomata.

In 1964 Dr. Roger Wyburn-Mason isolated free-living amoebae from all the tissues of patients suffering from rheumatoid disease. He then cultured the organisms in the laboratory to test the inhibitory effect of various substances. Those found to kill the amoebae were: metallic copper or copper salts, in minute traces; bile acids, in the concentration found in the small intestine; and anti-protozoal drugs including chloroquine and other 4-aminoquinolines, dehydroemetine, pentamidine, and compounds containing an imidazole group.[62]

AMOEBAE AS A CAUSE OF RHEUMATOID ARTHRITIS

All these substances have since been used in the treatment of active rheumatoid disease and may be clinically effective in abolishing activity in rhematoid disease. This indicates the presence of an amoeba in the affected tissues as the causative organism of the inflammation in subjects genetically sensitive to the organism.

HERXHEIMER REACTIONS

A number of drugs containing the anti-protozoal imidazole group produce *a Herxheimer reaction—a temporary exaggeration of symptoms followed by their lessening or disappearance.* This violent response in cases of rheumatoid disease indicates the presence of protozoa or gram-negative bacteria, which are acted on by these drugs.[30]

CHOICES IN MEDICATION

Many compounds containing the imidazole group were found by Dr. Wyburn-Mason to be effective against rheumatoid disease when all other treatments had failed. The activity of the disease was either abolished or did not return for a considerable period after treatment was stopped. The imidazole-containing compounds, including clotrimazole, appear to confer anti-protozoal activity against a spectrum of protozoa—including trichomonas, entamoeba hystolytica, giardia, and freeliving amoebae such as *Naegleria.* Since then he found that simpler, easier to use compounds containing the imidazole group were equally or more effective than clotrimazole. Metronidazole, tinidazole (which also contains a sulphone group in a side-chain), nimorazole, and ornidazole all demonstrate anti-protozoal properties and are highly effective against trichomonas, giardiasis, and entamoeba infections with practically no side effects. *Metronidazole is given three times daily for two to ten days,* whereas the other three substances are given in single weekly doses.

When treating rheumatoid disease, these compounds usually cause a brief exacerbation (worsening) of symptoms within 24 to 48 hours—with increased pain, swelling, and hotness in the affected joints and, often, in other joints not previously involved; other non-articular tissues may also show inflammatory changes. This reaction may be slight, or the patient may exhibit influenza-like symptoms—pain and stiffness in the neck, headache, and often a mild pyrexia and sweating, which may be drenching and nocturnal—and the sedimentation rate may rise.

When using the single-dose drugs this reaction usually followed within a day or so by another, followed by improvement in the arthritic symptoms. The reaction after each dose diminishes until, after 8 to 10 doses, it disappears. By this time the activity of the disease as judged by pain, heat, and swelling of joints seems to have disappeared. It was also found that *bursitis in the elbow, rheumatoid nodules, and palmar redness fade away.* Usually, the more severe the initial reaction, the better the final result.

When first using metronidazole, a dose of 250 mg to 500 mg is given three times daily for 10 days. During this time the patient may experience nausea and some anorexia.

During treatment none of these compounds produced changes in blood corpuscle, bone marrow, or liver function tests, and only rarely nausea. At the end of the treatment, the sedimentation rate tends to fall to normal. Bony cartilaginous changes are not improved, though adhesions may break down.

Example: A total of 60 cases of classical rheumatoid disease of varying duration, treated previously by a variety of anti-rheumatoid drugs, were given one of these imadazole substances, particularly the single-dose drugs. Tinidazole failed to produce any reaction whatsoever in one case, which later responded to metronidazole. One patient receiving metronidazole developed mild peripheral neuropathy after 6 weeks of treatment. Two other cases experienced the typical reaction at first, which then diminished and recurred again after repetition of the treatment, with no final improvement in condition. Both cases had been receiving steroids for 15 years or more and were severely afflicted with advanced osteoarthritic changes in the knees. The knee joints of one of these patients had been repeatedly aspirated yielding clear, slightly yellow fluid. After one dose of tinidazole, the knees swelled markedly and remained hot and painful, with free fluid in the joints. On aspiration both knees yielded thick, green, bacteriologically-sterile pus, indicating some action of the drug on an organism in the joint tissues.[36]

AMOEBAE INDENTIFIED AS A CAUSE OF RHEUMATOID ARTHRITIS

Overall it seems highly probable that *various species of free-living amoebae are the etiological agent of collagen-auto-immune diseases,* which show every gradation and combination with one another. *They are not due to a single organism but to a number of similar organisms.* Such a parasitic infection would explain the urticaria, asthma, and eosinophilia observed in many cases of collage or auto-immune diseases.

AMOEBAE CAUSING OTHER RELATED DISEASES

The list of chronic and degenerative diseases in which pathogenic protozoa have been found includes Paget's disease of the bone, ulcerative colitis, myasthenia gravis, arteritis, chronic pyelonephritis, some cases of diabetes, pericarditis, some cases of hepatitis and cirrhosis of the liver, uterine fibroids, ovarian cysts, and some types of malignancies such as lymphoma, leukemia, and Hodgkins disease. These organisms may also cause scleroderma, alopecia, vitaligo, melanoderma, eczema, psoriasis, and dermatitis herpetiformis of the skin; gingivitis, pyorrhea, and dental caries in the mouth; asthma and chronic bronchitis in the lungs; Parkinson's disease of the central nervous system; psychoses and gliomas.

Since these free-living amoebae are universally distributed in the environment, *reinfection in susceptible subjects is possible at any time.* The blood of healthy persons contains antibodies against these organisms; but in certain susceptible individuals, they may migrate from the gastrointestinal tract into the blood and then into the joints and other body tissues. Severe stress, injury, or illness may precipitate disease by lowering general tissue resistance and permit the spread or localization of protozoa which under other circumstances might not cause symptoms.[62]

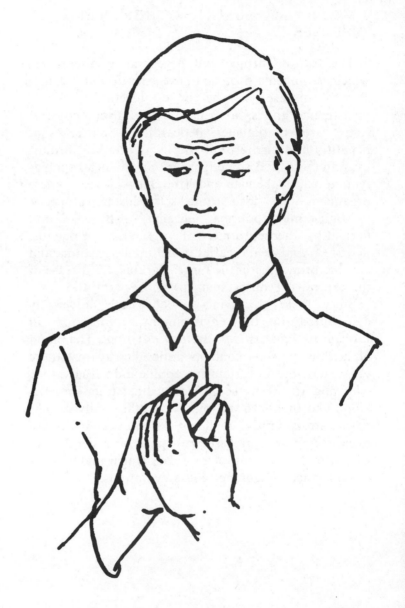

STRESS PREDISPOSES

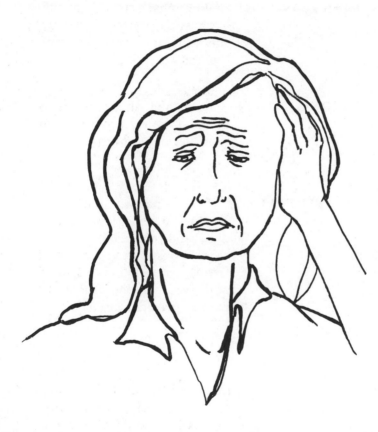

TO ARTHRITIS

Table 6

INDIRECT CAUSES OF ARTHRITIS

STRESS   Emotional strain, mental exhaustion, physical fatigue, illness, injury, overwork, grief.

ENVIRONMENTAL   Cold and damp weather, polluted water, contaminated food, famine, poverty.

OCCUPATIONAL   Toxic metals: aluminum, mercury, arsenic, lead, certain dyes and chemicals, insecticides, pesticides, chemical food preservatives and additives, smog, fumes of paints, plastics, varnishes.

INTERNAL   Allergies, food and vitamin deficiencies, mineral deficiencies, chronic infections, metabolic disorders, hormone deficiencies, premature aging, arteriosclerosis, drug and alcohol addiction, tobacco smoking, sensitivity or intolerance to medicines.

CHAPTER 6

STRESS AND OTHER INDIRECT CAUSES

Stress includes all external (environmental) and internal (mental and emotional) factors that put "pressure" on the patient. Every individual is affected by different stress situations, and every individual reacts differently to the same stresses.

The medical literature once claimed there is no such disease as psychologically-produced, or "psychosomatic," arthritis. There is no evidence of a "rheumatoid personality," and treatment of psychological factors does not seem to influence the outcome of the disease. But there is physiological proof that *stress can predispose to arthritis by making a patient more susceptible to the disease.*

However, arthritis can occur without any known emotional or mental stress. Juvenile rheumatoid arthritis (JRA), or Still's disease, occurs in infants and children and has the same clinical manifestations as rheumatiod arthritis in adults. But it is rare or absent in children who live in the stress situations of war, famine, and poverty; nor is the incidence of rheumatoid arthritis in adults increased by these factors—the most stressful conditions under which many people must survive.

But if an individual living under severe stress acquires poor eating habits, he may develop nutritional deficiencies and the factors which apparently cause rheumatoid arthritis are more likely to result in an active disease.

Nutritionists know *that stress interferes with appetite, digestion, food choices and absorption, and basic dietary patterns.* Through the thalamic centers in the brain and the sympathetic nervous system, stress controls the glands of internal secretion—particularly the thyroid, adrenals, and pituitary—and generates inhibitory nerve impulses to the circulatory and immunological systems of the body. Such disturbance in the nervous system produces biological changes in the body which affect bone and joint metabolism. The individual is weakened and becomes more susceptible to arthritis as well as such diseases as peptic ulcers, hypertension, anemia, hypothyroidisms, adrenal deficiency, and even cancer.

EXTERNAL STRESS

External (environmental) stress comes from climate, living conditions, economic and social positions in life, occupation, marital problems (particularly divorce or incompatibility), child care and discipline, illnesss or death of a loved one, polluted air and water, poor diet, vitamin and mineral deficiency, lack of exercise, dissatisfaction with personal goals, and general unhappiness.

Some patients find that suffering from arthritis "rewards" them with more love, care, and attention from family and friends than they ever had when they were well. Such a patient does not want to "give up" his disease and return to the previous situation of good health and the neglect of his family and friends. So he rejects therapy, even though he does not consciously accept this reason for his failure to attempt recovery from arthritis.

He may receive disability income or insurance benefits that would be forfeited if he recovered. He might have to return to an unpleasant, unsatisfying, and stressful job if he was less physically handicapped. He would "rather have arthritis."

On the other hand, he may believe that arthritis is

punishment for real or imaginary sins, bad habits, or self-neglect. He is racked with guilt and nurses his arthritis symptoms as a sort of self-flagellation. He prefers to "suffer" rather than get well, accepting medication only to relieve the pain or to tranquilize himself into tolerating the discomfort and disability.

Another patient who was strong and healthy before the onset of arthritis may feel that, if he was really strong enough, he could make the disease go away and becomes depressed when he cannot voluntarily "will" it into remission. He considers a thorough program of arthritis management a waste of time and money.

INTERNAL STRESS

Internal (mental and emotional) stress may be triggered by an outside event or circumstance that continues after the original cause has disappeared. Such stress factors can often be alleviated with psychological or religious counseling.

If people could learn from childhood how to cope with stress, they probably would have better health and the incidence of arthritis would decline. "Getting arthritis" is one way certain people respond to stress. By learning to understand and recognize their responses to stress, arthritis patients can live longer, have fewer symptoms, get better results from treatment, more readily adapt to any residual disabilities, and accept the recommendations of their medical advisors.

Because of the role of the stress on individuals, arthritis treatment must include emphasis on emotional factors. *Patients* should not feel that they have no control over their treatment. They *must be assured that they can actively participate in their treatment and consequently make a more rapid, complete recovery.*

THE "ARTHRITIS" PERSONALITY

Certain personality types in their reaction to stress seem predisposed to arthritis. These patients display repression, denial, and depression. They have been unuable to cope with some important phase of their lives—personal or family relationships, employment, religious conflict, loss of a loved one. They are rigid in their dietary routines, the lack of physical activity, and dependence on certain medications.

Patients who make good recoveries from arthritis are emotionally stable, try to be physically active, are flexible in their attitudes, and are able to learn from the physician and the medical staff. *Patients with a strong belief in themselves, who set goals of accomplishment, and who believe in their improvement or recovery respond best to treatment.*
The hopeless outlook of recovery defeats many arthritis patients. They have gone from doctor to doctor, from clinic to clinic, and have taken dozens of different drugs. Nothing seems to help and they continue to get worse. Many patients are pessimistic, discouraged, and unenthusiastic when they first come to the Desert Arthritis Medical Clinic. They believe they can never get well. *When* such *patients learn to follow a new pattern of life and to actively participate in their own care and treatment, they usually improve and achieve a remission of their disease,* with complete recovery in some cases.[10]

OTHER INDIRECT CAUSES

METABOLIC DISORDERS

Hormonal imbalance such as arising from menopause and other glandular deficiencies of the thyroid, adrenals, and pancreas may interfere with metabolism and contribute to the cause of arthritis, particularly in the disease osteoporosis. Hyperthyroidism, hypothyroidism, gout with excessive uric acid, chronic kidney disease, and even intestinal disturbances such as diarrhea and constipation may interfere with bone metabolism. Hormone deficiency can be partly offset by improvement in nutrition and health, but often actual hormone replacement is necessary. *Post-menopausal women may need supplemental estrogen for calcium replenishment of osteoporotic bone.* For osteoporosis and arthritis patients, the risk of cancer aggravation by hormone treatment is much less than the certainty of increased pain, deformity, and disability due to protein and ovarian deficiencies.

Example: An often neglected area in the search for factors influencing arthritis are the intestines. The medical workup of arthritis patients in the United States is deficient because both physicians and patients have a distaste for stool examinations, and most laboratories are unable to perform complete stool examinations. In a fine hospital in France, every patient has a thorough stool examination and a third or more have been found with some disease or deficiency requiring medical treatment. Chronic bacterial and virus infections, ova and parasites, occult blood, and poorly digested food products indicate disorders which require further investigation and correction.

Gastrointestinal disturbances are often found in arthritis patients, which may explain why *some popular herbs and food extracts such as yucca, alfalfa, and herb teas seem to help so many of them.* Fasting, enemas, and the almost discarded procedure of colonic irrigations benefit some arthritis patients through a thorough cleansing of the lower intestinal tract. However, the frequent use of anti-acids, laxatives and cathartics interferes with digestion and normal bowel absorption and can contribute to the arthritis syndrome.

PREMATURE AGING

The difference between a person's chronological age (years) and his biological age (health) is the amount of vitality he has. *Healthy people are actually "younger than their years" and live longer* than those in ill health. Poor dietary habits are a major factor in premature old age, which is expecially significant in the development of osteoarthritis. *Overeating and obesity can be just as damaging to the joints as undereating and nutritional deficiency.* Other factors in premature aging are accidents, illness, and chronic disease; smoking, drinking alcohol, and the use of drugs in excess; environmental and emotional stress; overwork; and chronic poor sleep habits.

ARTERIOSCLEROSIS

Arteriosclerosis results from deposits of excess fatty substances in the arteries. These deposits interfere with circulation to the bones and joints and reduces their metabolism and oxygen supply, causing degeneration, and finally degenerative arthritis. *Normal human cartilage should last more than 100 years; but once worn away or destroyed, it cannot be biologically replaced by healing processes.* The aim of every arthritis treatment is to preserve and protect the remaining cartilage surfaces in all affected joints.[57]

HEALING BY FAITH AND BY PRAYER

Most physicians believe that *stress* may cause or aggravate arthritis. Many arthritis patients have tensions, anxieties and fears to a greater extent than healthy persons. Because these diseases can result in severe and progressive disability only cancer produces more mental and emotional concerns than the onset of an attack of arthritis.

Treating and relieving this worry and nervous strain is one of the duties of physicians. So very often this is temporarily accomplished by prescriptions of other drugs, tranquilizers or mood elevators, without getting to the cause of the problem. Supplying medical information about the patients' diseases and enlisting their cooperation to "Fight Back" are ways patients are helped to overcome their troubled minds. Spiritual and emotional support are other resources which can be utilized in most cases.

In every primitive society there have been, and are today, certain persons to whom is attributed the "Power of Healing." They are know as "Faith Healers, Witchdoctors," or "Curanderos" who by their prayers, incantations and various ministrations appear to effect many "cures." Many of these appear to be for patients suffering with arthritis and the relief of arthritis pain and stiffness is frequently seen and can be verified.

It must be recognized that some of these "miraculous cures" may be from disorders of the body which are purely "functional" - in the patient's mind but not subject to his understanding and control. The "miracle workers" often take credit for healing which is already occurring through natural processes and the restorative functions of the human body.

Medical science is aware of the close relationship of disorders of the mind and emotional disturbances to physical illnesses. Anxiety and depression can produce poor health through lack of rest and sleep, from malnutrition, by lack of activity and exercise and from "nervous exhaustion" and overwork. These are factors in susceptibility to arthritis.

On the other hand strong mental and emotional stimuli in a positive manner release beneficial hormones into the blood stream, the endomorphins from the central nervous system and substances from the adrenal glands, which relieve pain and muscle spasm and improve circulation to affected joints.

Healing of the mind and spirit has been shown to have anatomical and biochemical bases for the improvement they achieve in relieving physical diseases in addition to the benefits from the purely mental, emotional and spiritual aspects of such treatments.

Some of these "healings" by faith and prayer appear to happen "in an instant", others occur more slowly, but almost always they seem to take place more rapidly than could be accomplished by conventional medical treatment.

The Bible relates that one of the powers given to Christ's disciples was the "Gift of Healing" of both physical and mental ills. This requires the use of prayer, the laying on of hands, and often the symbolic anointing with oil.

In this century there has been a revival of interest and practice of healing by faith and prayer in the Protestant and Catholic churches, beginning first in the Episcopal, long considered very conservative, and spreading now to other denominations. Every congregation which has a healing ministry can relate many success stories of their accomplishments as well as plausible explantions for their failures.

As a boy I was taken to healing services in Denver, Colorado held by Amiee Semple MacPherson, accompanied by my father who as a medical missionary to Latin America was both a medical doctor and a Baptist minister. We saw many "cures" and some he was able to medically verify.

More recently the late Katherine Kuhlman and the modern fundamentalist television ministers such as Oral Roberts have publicly demonstrated that many hundreds, perhaps thousands, of sick and handicapped persons can and will be healed in a way that medical science cannot adequately explain. They call upon the powers of God to heal the lame and the afflicted whom we with our medical skills still cannot cure.

As an open-minded and scientifically trained physician I strongly recommend that every patient with chronic arthritis and progressive rheumatoid disease find spiritual as well as medical help while seeking physical improvement and recovery. In this search, similar to the finding of the best available doctor, family and friends should help and recommend ministers, and churches, who are knowledgeable and sympathetic to healing by faith and prayer. For we all know that in every sick body there may be a sick mind or spirit seeking help and understanding.

Being raised in a doctor's family and as a physician I have been fortunate in being able to observe over fifty years of medical progress and the acceleration of scientific knowledge about the human body which has been a phenomenon of this century. But when we realize how much is yet to be learned we must be humble and forever seeking new truths.

While I have respect for every man and his right to the belief and worship of his choice I can only report that as a Christian with a firm belief in Jesus Christ I have a faith that has sustained me in all of the problems and dangers of life and that has helped me in the practice of medicine. Whatever success I have had in treating patients, making small but new medical discoveries, and understanding the mysteries of the human body I attribute to this help that has come to me through my religion.

For this reason I can recommend, just as strongly as I advise physical treatment, that the arthritis patient with the help of his family and friends undertake the search for spiritual and mental healing that can only come with building a faith in God and learning to pray. The spiritual forces can give new and better meaning to life, even in the presence of suffering and physical disability.

There is no real conflict between medical science and true religion. Both are seeking answers to what is still unknown, but what will someday be known, in a spiritual world and life in which there is no death and no disease.

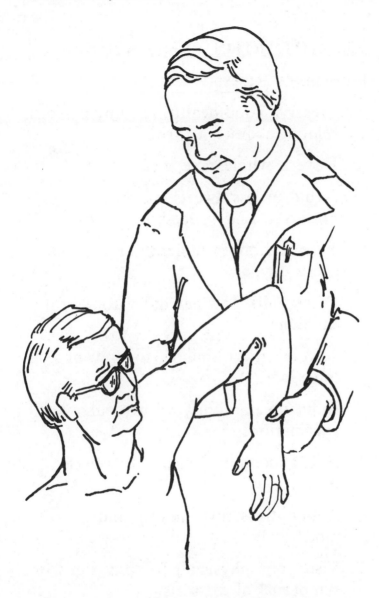

JOINT EXAMINATIONS SHOULD BE THOROUGH

Table 7
ARTHRITIS PREVENTION

Ten Simple Rules:

1. Preserve good health. Healthy persons seldom acquire arthritis.

2. Have a wholesome diet.

3. Avoid excess sweets, starches, preserved and processed foods.

4. Take a vitamin-mineral supplement every day.

5. Drink milk and eat dairy foods for calcium.

6. Take extra vitamin C to prevent infections.

7. Build up immunity with regular vaccinations.

8. Avoid alcohol, tobacco and toxic drugs.

9. Avoid stress, live quietly and moderately.

10. Visit your physician for any signs or symptoms of arthritis.

CHAPTER 7

THE PREVENTION OF ARTHRITIS

TO INSURE THAT YOUR JOINTS LAST 100 YEARS you must start the prevention of arthritis before you are born. Your mother must not smoke tobacco or marijuana, drink alcohol sparingly or not at all, and take great care in her diet and exercise. She should be immunized against the common virus diseases, particularly rubella and poliomyelitis. And she should avoid harmful radiation, UNNECESSARY x-rays and electrical treatments.

The mother's diet is most important. It should contain an adequate volume of protein, particularly fish, poultry and the dairy foods. Carbohydrates should come chiefly from fresh fruit and vegetables and the whole grain cereals. Adequate fats are present in milk, cheese, butter and five to ten eggs a week. Of course, we recommend the highest quality milk, Certified Raw Milk, but unfortunately due to misinformed health departments this is not available in most parts of the country.

Exercise is most necessary for the expectant mother who is striving to have the most healthy and normal baby possible. The circulation of the body, blood to the muscles and joints, and even the flow to the brain is increased by regular physical activity. Walking, swimming and bicycle riding are best. Golf and tennis are fine for young mothers. And don't give up sexual exercise until the doctor decides term is near. During the last months and weeks of pregnancy regular exercise will help baby move about in the uterus, avoiding deformities of the extremities and assisting proper positioning for delivery.

SUPPLEMENTAL VITAMINS AND MINERALS are necessary during the pregnancy, as it is almost impossible to consume a "normal well-balanced diet" containing enough of these elements without gaining too much body weight. Many well balanced pre-natal formulae are on the market, or a therapeutic vitamin and mineral combination can be chosen. We recommend the mother take two of these a day, as there is often some loss in digestion and assimilation with the intestinal changes during pregnancy, and two of these vitamin/mineral capsules is far below the toxic dose.

TO PREVENT ARTHRITIS the nutrition of the child is very important, especially during the growth period and to the end of adolescence. Snack and convenience foods have become to play such a large role in the eating habits of most children, especially between meals, after school and in the evening while studying or watching television, that vitamin and mineral supplements are necessary—from birth to about 16 years of age in girls and to 18 years of age in boys—the time of most rapid bone growth and development.

"Everyone knows" how important vitamin D is in the bottle fed infant and growing child to prevent rickets. Yet so many young mothers stop the vitamin drops when bottle feeding stops and neglect to continue their children on liquid syrup vitamins or chewable vitamins until they willingly swallow pills. As a result this generation of children is replete with flat chests, narrow jaws and crowded teeth requiring orthodontic care, spinal and postural abnormalities, and poorly developed and poorly aligned hips, knees and feet. These are the joints which will be more susceptible to arthritis later in life.

STARCHES AND SWEETS are the greatest threats to good bone and joint development in the growing child. If all the starches were from grains and vegetables and all the sweets from fruits there would be no problem. But white sugar, white flour and the common fats and oils used in cooking seem to have an affinity for each other—in candy, cakes, pies, cookies, commercial ice creams, white bread and sugar coated cereals. Soft drinks contain not only sugar, or synthetic sweeteners, but acids and preservatives that are not only detrimental of themselves but take away the child's appetite for better foods.

MILK IS THE BEST SOURCE OF CALCIUM and two to three glasses a day from infancy to old age is a good nutritional practice. With children, however, some discretion must be exercised to keep them from drinking too much, which would be over one quart (four glasses) a day, or drinking too much at mealtimes—thus decreasing their appetites and capacities for other foods.

Between the ages of about 10 to 14 in girls and 12 to 16 years of age in boys, drinking too much milk, more than two glasses a day, may lead to excess growth in height and very tall and thin children due to the growth hormones in cows milk—which makes a heifer from a calf in one year. On the other hand, the hormones in certified raw milk will increase the size of the breasts in girls and in women of any age—a "plus" that those with "flat chests" may appreciate.

DURING ADULT LIFE continuing to drink milk, avoiding the sweet and starchy foods, restricting fats and keeping body weight within normal limits is "arthritis prevention". A mineral and vitamin supplement should be taken regularly, and we say "because one is good, two is better" each and every day. Smoking is very bad for the joints, as stated in the chapter on solanines. Regular exercise, at least 20 minutes a day three times a week, is about the minimum which will maintain good circulation in the muscles and joints. Avoiding heavy lifting, not over 40 pounds repeatedly nor over 80 pounds occasionally, will protect the back. Sitting, standing or riding more than two hours at a time can be harmful if it is done every day. "Rest breaks" or "activity breaks" every hour or two for five to ten minutes is protection against bad posture, poor circulation and joint problems.

ELDERLY PERSONS should have no joint diseases if they have maintained lifelong patterns of good health and have been able to avoid serious illnesses, chronic infections, allergies and joint injuries.

THERE IS NO ARTHRITIS DUE TO OLD AGE. A moderate stiffness and some muscular weakness and atrophy may occur with reduced physical activity. I have examined patients from ninety to one hundred years of age who have had no arthritis. They frequently come from rural America or a foreign country where they were raised on natural foods and did physical work in their youth. You have only one set of joints in your life. Protect them.

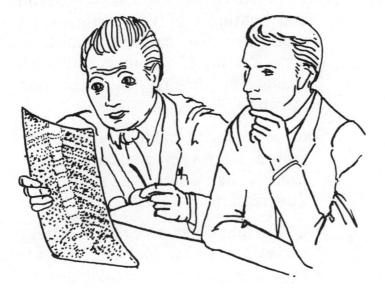

X-RAYS ARE NECESSARY TO AN ACCURATE DIAGNOSIS

Table 8
THE TREATMENT PROGRAM

To recover from arthritis you must also regain good health.

1. Have a personal physician, in family practice or internal medicine. Rely on him for restoration of your health and treatment of your arthritis. (A rheumatologist can be called in consultation. The primary physician should be health and nutrition oriented).

2. Start a complete medical and health record. Keep a personal copy and see that your doctor has all the information.

3. Ask your physician to order a dietary survey and a hair analysis. Tests for food allergies or cytotoxic testing may be indicated.

4. Keep a diary or log of all medications and treatments.

5. Read all you can about your disease. An informed patient will become the "recovered patient".

CHAPTER 8

THE TREATMENT PROGRAM

RECOVERY FROM ARTHRITIS is the goal; an active endeavor which you must initiate, pursue with your doctor, explore the many choices of treatment and learn to be become a well informed patient. No person ill with arthritis ever improves or recovers by medical management alone. The patient must WANT to get WELL. Does this sound strange? Would anyone with a painful and disabling rheumatic disease WANT to stay SICK? Yes, some of those afflicted with one of these diseases may find that the attention they get and help from their family and loved ones is so much greater that what they received while well that they "continue to enjoy being an invalid". Others may have disability payments for being off work, early retirement, avoiding employment which is disliked, or similar motives which consciously or unconsiously interferes with their desire to get well.

There must be a conscious determination to FIGHT BACK AGAINST ARTHRITIS, a *"will to win"*, a desire to learn as much as possible about their type of disease, and to use—not only drugs, or perhaps no drugs at all in many cases, but each and every method and treatment available until the best and right ones are found which work for you. That is why this book is full of new and different remedies which have been tested and found to be successful for large numbers of patients. There is no fixed rule or magic formula as to which ones should be done first. That depends on you, your type of disease, your freedom to travel if necessary, your doctor's advice and your financial circumstances.

There are estimates of more than 30 million patients

with arthritis in the United States. We would like all of
them to know the possibilities of recovery and have the
hope and inspiration to find improvement and a cure.
We can only reach a small number of them with this
book. But this information will also reach hundreds,
perhaps thousands, of physicians. And the medical
knowledge and experiences recorded here may
encourage them to take a broader view of arthritis
treatment and be brave enough to be innovative, even
if it means being "controversial" for the sake of their
patients.

A. YOUR GENERAL HEALTH

For thousands of years the world has undergone
changes in human and animal life, in vegetation, and in
the weather—evolution resulting from *the "balance of
nature."* Some are caused by natural events such as
fire, earthquake, storms, and floods. Others are man-
made: cutting down the forests, damming rivers,
building cities on former farm lands, and the ravages of
war.

Naturalists, environmentalists, and public health
authorities are concerned with changes in the balance
of nature brought on by pesticides, air and water
pollution, impure foods, and dangerous drugs—all
which can enter the body and have a harmful effect on
our health. To overcome these adverse environmental
factors, governmental, health, industrial, and business
factions are engaged in research programs to reduce
the toxic wastes produced by our civilized world. The
concern of the public shows an increasing interest
through the news media, books, and journals.

THE BALANCE OF NATURE

Every human being enjoys *a personal "balance of nature"* which produces and maintains good health. The functions of a healthy person depend on the balance of nature being maintained between physical, mental, and spiritual well-being. The strength of these internal forces keeps the body healthy and well, even against the external, adverse forces so often present in the environment.

Better than 99% of all newborns have a normal, healthy start in life. A number of rare diseases and deformities affecting the newborn are being reduced through medical study and treatment. Since the human infant is devoid of the instincts of self-preservation found in other species, the well-being of a child must be preserved by good nutrition, a clean environment, and tender loving care. Immunization against common childhood diseases is required for good child care.

MAINTAINING GOOD HEALTH

Three necessities of life contribute to good health: *nutrition, exercise,* and *rest.* Without these the span of life is shortened and *premature old age* and *physical degeneration result.*

•NUTRITION

Abundant *natural foods appropriate to the latitude and climate exist in every area of the world* and are nutritionally compatible with the good health of those living there.

Fish and seals in the arctic are high in protein and fat necessary for cold days and long winter nights. The abundant fruits of the tropics are high in carbohydrates as well as *vitamins C and B-complex, which are not stored in the body but used up by exercise in the hot sun.*

Each individual requires a different balance of protein, carbohydrates, fats, minerals, and vitamins according to *age, physical activity,* and *climate. Food deficiencies cause many types of illness as the lack of vital nutrients lowers resistance and predisposes to infectious diseases from viruses, bacteria, fungi, and protozoa. Good nutrition is the first step in preventing disease.*

•EXERCISE

The bones, muscles, lungs, and heart require physical activity and exercise to maintain good health. The bones become stronger the longer they carry the body's weight. The muscles are totally dependent on regular use and exercise to maintain their strength and flexibility. Circulation to the brain, heart, lungs, and internal organs is dependent partially on physical activity. The volume, oxygen content, and rate of flow of blood is increased with exercise and decreased by inactivity.

•REST

Sleep is the most profound state of rest and the body cannot go without it for very long. During sleep physical and mental activity is at minimum, allowing the internal organs to digest and absorb food and make it available for the repair and replacement of body cells.

Even *the teeth,* among the hardest and strongest of the body's structures, must have a fresh new supply of calcium about once a year and require the natural cellular activities of a healthy mouth.

Rest is also necessary for calm and peaceful thinking, reading, and mental activity which contributes to a perons's sense of security, physical comfort, and ability to work and function efficiently.

SPIRITUAL HEALTH

The spiritual forces in life, including conscience and the knowledge of good and evil, are just as important but harder to identify. They are present in the oneness felt with nature and the beauty of the world around us; they are the inspiration for great ideas, creations in music, art, and literature, and new discoveries and inventions. *Spiritual forces also are demonstrated in the associations of man with one another,* in the love that bonds families together, and in patriotism and love of country. The communion of the mind and spirit with God in meditation and prayer contributes to the balance of nature and the spiritual forces in life.

The Bible says: "Be not decieved, God is not mocked. Whatsoever a man soweth, that shall he also reap." This applies to the balance of nature in the body. The lack of good nutrition, overwork, harmful habits, the use of alcohol, tobacco, and the abuse of drugs upset the balance of nature and will produce ill health, disease, and physical degeneration.

The prevention and treatment of arthritis is based on recognizing and applying these principles to preserving and restoring the balance of nature.

B. YOUR DOCTOR

The patient-physician relationship must be one of confidence, patience, and continued cooperation. They should both be satisfied with the diagnosis, course of treatment, and remission or recovery achieved.

The majority of arthritis patients are treated by their family physicians or specialists in internal medicine. Rheumatologists, who specialize in rheumatism and arthritis, treat only about 15 percent of arthritis patients—the most severe and disabled. But, they may see more severe arthritis patients in a day than the average internist or general practitioner may see in a month.

Whatever his specialty the physician must inform, educate, persuade, assist, and supervise his patient with *every known measure to control the disease and restore to health.* His assistance is necessary for basic diagnostic studies and to begin medical treatment. But if he is not certain of the diagnosis he should send the patient to another doctor, or the patient should ask for a referral.

For convenience as well as better medical care, most clinics will refer patients to an arthritis specialist for further examinations, laboratory tests, and x-rays.

This is not "passing the buck." *Both patients and physicians are seeking a "second opinion" more often these days*—especially when the diagnosis is uncertain; or when the outcome of the disease may be serious, chronic, or critical; or when the physician has neither the knowledge or resources to carry out effective treatment. The patient should not feel embarrassed asking for a referral, and the physician should not hesitate in recommending such a procedure. He should also forward to the consulting physician copies of the patient's medical history, all laboratory reports, the original x-rays with their interpretations, and, if possible, his personal assessment of the patient's case. The consultant should refer the patient back to his physician for treatment.

THE COUNSELOR

The average physician cannot afford to spend 4 or 5 hours with each patient discussing such general aspects of health as diet, living habits, stress, vitamins, etc. Likewise, the patient could not afford to pay for so much of the doctor's time, nor would any insurance company reimburse the patient for these services.

Consequently, a *trained counselor* is often called upon to discuss these things with the patient, to listen to his special problems and fears in the routine management of his disease, and to answer general questions the patient may be hesitant to ask his doctor for fear of "wasting his time."

Arthritis counselors are usually arthritis patients who have recovered or adapted to their residual handicaps. They are perhaps best suited to advise an arthritis patient on his personal participation in his home therapy.

Social interactions between patients are also important because they learn from each other. They benefit from meeting and sharing experiences with patients who may have more serious forms of the disease but who have made good recoveries.

UNSATISFACTORY RESULTS

If some therapies fail the patient should not feel personally responsible, nor should the physician feel inadequate. All patients and cases of arthritis are different, and a certain amount of clinical trials are necessary to find the combination of treatments that gives the best results. This may take a good deal of time, expense, and effort; but *the final result, recovery from arthritis, is worth all the costs.*

This attitude applies directly to *arthritis,* where so *many drugs now being used only partly relieve the symptoms but do not cure the disease.* A patient "cured" of active arthritis may have some residual stiffness, limitation of joint motion, or weakness due to joint damage; but he should have *no pain, swelling, tenderness, or inflammation,* and the disease should not be progressive or getting worse.

The "total approach" to arthritis management involves treating the patient as a "whole person." Every aspect of his physical, psychological, social, and economic condition should be considered in seeking a diagnosis and in treating his disease. This "wholistic" treatment requires the expertise of specialists in medicine, physical therapy, applied nutrition, and orthopedic surgery.

THE PATIENT'S RESPONSIBILITY

The goal of every patient is to get well. The physician can supply the diagnosis and medical treatment; but some other measures are under the patient's control: climate and environment: diet, vitamins, and minerals; exercise and physical therapy.

Non-conventional treatments—such as arthritis vaccine, special diets, vitamin and mineral therapy, yucca extract, esterene, anti-protozoal drugs—may or may not be approved by the patient's personal physician and are available only from certain limited sources. Then the patient must decide for himself which treatments he will try.

As soon as the patient realizes he *can* get well and live a happier, more useful life, he will begin to improve. He actively participates in his treatment and his body cooperates to resist the disease. He must learn to analyze and dispose of the stress factors in his life, to engage in physical exercise for his physical and emotional well-being, and to improve his general health through diet, vitamin and mineral supplements, and physical therapy.

C. YOUR MEDICAL RECORDS

In seeking a definite diagnosis, the patient should request copies of all medical records, x-rays, and laboratory reports for his own use. Even though the x-rays and original records remain the property of the examining physician or hospital, the patient is entitled to their use or should be furnished copies.

Personal medical records are invaluable to the arthritis patient. He should maintain a file to accumulate these reports during the treatment of his disease and for the rest of his life. The family physician may keep this record for the patient, who should request that copies be forwarded to subsequent doctors when necessary.

Physicians, radiologists, and hospitals commonly forward to the consulting physician x-ray films only and not the reports. But the radiologist's interpretation is often more valuable than the films themselves and provides another opinion to check against his own. Therefore, when authorizing a transfer of records, the patient should request that copies of the radiologist's report accompany the films.

A patient's complete medical record should contain the following items:

1. MEDICAL HISTORY. Past medical history including information regarding all illnesses, injuries, or operations previous to the onset of arthritis; any illness or injury which preceded the onset of arthritis, including which joints were involved; initial examinations or treatments; progress of the disease;

continued treatments; drugs prescribed and taken (names, amounts, dates) and any other medical conditions seemingly unrelated to arthritis. Note that reactions from some medications may occur weeks or months after first administered, particularly after prolonged use.

2. PHYSICAL EXAMINATION. Arthritis involvement should include descriptions of the joints, range of motion, presence of heat, swelling, and tenderness. The general physical examination should pay special attention to heart, lungs, eyes, muscles, and circulation as some arthritis syndromes affect these areas. Descriptions of body systems should be complete—with positive, negative, or normal findings.

3. LABORATORY TESTS. The minimum necessary are complete blood count (CBC), hematocrit, sedimentation rate, blood chemistry panel (including tests for diabetes, gout, and the mineral levels of calcium and phosphorus), rheumatoid serology tests, RA factor and urinalysis. More extensive blood tests may be indicated later depending on the probable clinical diagnosis.

4. X-RAY EXAMINATIONS. Joints: the most involved, (especially the hands), weight bearing joints, and usually the spine. Chest: often reveals old or active lung disease. The lateral chest x-ray is a good survey of arthritis in the thoracic spine.

5. DRUG TREATMENT. Dosages; duration of treatment; reactions (both favorable and unfavorable); any intolerances, allergies, sensibilities, or evidences of toxicity.

6. UNRELATED CONDITIONS. Physical handicaps or non-arthritic diseases, especially allergies, infections, chronic conditions, general poor health.

7. PROBABLE DIAGNOSIS. No case of arthritis should be treated just as "arthritis." A definite classification, or your doctor's "clinical impression," is necessary to select the proper treatment.

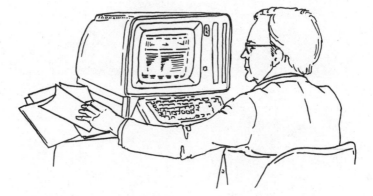

**GET A COMPUTERIZED PRINT-OUT OF
YOUR CLINICAL LABORATORY TESTS
FINDINGS**

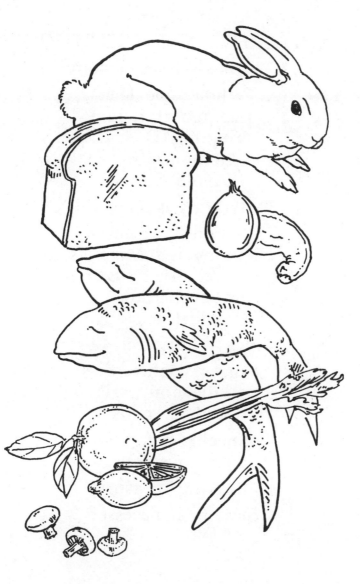

PROTEIN FOODS
BUILD NEW TISSUES

Table 9
ARTHRITIS AND NUTRITION
1. Arthritis is Preventable

Wholesome Diet
Adequate Calcium
Vitamins D & C
Immunization
Avoid Stress

2. Arthritis is Treatable

Good Nutrition
Vitamins and Minerals
Necessary Drugs
Vaccination
Physical Therapy

3. Much Arthritis is Curable

Correct Deficiencies
in diet, minerals
and vitamins

Specific drugs for
infectious causes

Physical measures

Surgery if necessary

CHAPTER 9

NUTRITION AND ARTHRITIS

WILL SPECIAL DIETS HELP ARTHRITIS? No field of arthritis therapy is as controversial as the role of nutrition in the prevention and in the treatment of rheumatoid disease.

Every person has an individual attitude towards food which is a result of combining his heredity, his family, race, culture and his environment.

For Example: Dr. Collin H. Dong, M.D., the author of the book, "New Hope for the Arthritic", is a famous and well respected physician in the San Francisco area who has helped many patients with his diet recommendations. But because he is Chinese, and because this race has less arthritis than Anglo-Saxons, his diets are much like the basic foods of the Chinese people—no red meat, lots of fish and poultry, no dairy products, etc. And while this is a healthy diet it has no direct relation to arthritis, as a recent clinical study has shown.

A bewildering number of diets have been extolled for arthritis. Many of these contradict each other— vegetarian, high protein, no milk, fasting, high calcium, low calcium high vitamin, no nucleoproteins, no nightshade foods, no processed foods, no artificial preservatives or additives, etc. Yet the good intentions and personal experiences of their proponents can not be questioned. Some of these diets have helped some patients, somewhere, sometime.

The dietary program recommended in this book has been developed and tested in the Desert Arthritis Medical Clinic and has the accumulated wisdom and experience of twenty years in treating all types of arthritis diseases.

ARTHRITIS DOES NOT COME ON OVERNIGHT, and no change in the diet will work an overnight "cure". However, the proper combination of the best "body-building" foods and the elimination of the allergic and low quality foods will improve health and help to FIGHT BACK AGAINST ARTHRITIS.

THERE IS NO SINGLE BEST DIET for all arthritis patients. Every individual reacts to foods in his own, unique way. And the needs of each body depends on age, weight, sex, health, physical activity, the disease process present, and even on such factors as geography and the weather.

In the next two chapters the TREATMENT OF ARTHRITIS WITH GOOD NUTRITION will be discussed in detail. Two principles should become general knowledge—Arthritis is Preventable, and Arthritis is Treatable. The history and background for these facts are unique and probably controversial.

A. ARTHRITIS IS PREVENTABLE. *No one in good nutritional health develops rheumatoid arthritis or osteoarthritis.*

The *rheumatoid arthritis patient* usually has a diet deficient in proteins and vitamins. He is nervous, tense, anxious, and over-active; he is not getting enough rest or the right kinds of food; he has poor resistance to infection, often with a past history of many chronic inflammatory or infectious diseases.

The osteoarthritis patient is usually middle-aged or elderly and overweight. He is often poorly nourished on a high carbohydrate diet which is dominant in refined flour, sweets, and fats and deficient in protein, vitamins, and enzymes—and has been so for months or years prior to the onset of his disease.

Although arthritis is a family of many types of diseases diet and nutrition are common factors in both their cause and treatment. *Nutritional deficiency makes an individual susceptible to arthritis,* and good nutrition is the best and only method for its prevention. Arthritis occurs only in patients with inadequate joint nutrition whether caused by dietary deficiency, stress, illness, disease, injury, poor circulation, or nerve injury.

B. ARTHRITIS IS TREATABLE. It can be arrested and is often curable. Most arthritis patients do not know that nutrition is such an important factor in the cause and treatment of their disease. They are often satisfied with the quality of their dietary intake in the same way that many people are "satisfied" with their religion or way of life. *But good nutrition and the correction of dietary deficiencies* is *necessary for the successful treatment of all types of arthritis.* Some types of arthritis can be relieved or "cured" by therapeutic nutrition alone, but therapy for rheumatoid arthritis and osteoarthritis must include correction of metabolic as well as nutritional deficiencies.

When the physician is not educated in the value of good nutrition, then *the patient must take the initiative to learn his own personal needs and to supply them.* The use of applied nutrition in the treatment of arthritis differs from the usual medical treatment routines in that it will produce improvement and even recovery in many early cases.

C. THE HISTORY OF APPLIED NUTRITION

About 26 years ago Dr. Joseph E. Risser, the world famous orthopedic surgeon and scoliosis specialist, introduced me to "applied nutrition." He found that growth and development of the spine is influenced by the diet of his patients. A lack of calcium in the diet or hydrochloric acid in the stomach delays bone growth and repair after fusion operations; while an excess of carbohydrates, especially *refined white flour and white sugar products, has a similar retarding action on bone and joint development.*

Under Dr. Risser's sponsorship I joined the American Academy of Applied Nutrition (now the *International College of Applied Nutrition*), an organization of physicians, dentists and scientists in related fields who study human nutrition and use this knowledge in their practices.

Academy member Francis A. Pottinger, Jr., was instrumental in making *Certified raw milk* available in the Los Angeles area, which has been invaluable to thousands of patients—especially crippled children and those with bone and joint disorders. He produced experimental arthritis in cats by feeding them pasteurized milk and cooked meat, then cured them with natural raw milk and raw meat.[46]

Michael A. Walsh, D.Sc., a famous biochemist and a leader in the Academy, developed the *computerized diet analysis* used today to record and evaluate the nutritional intake of patients and provide guidance for dietary and food supplement prescriptions.[45]

NUTRITION AND POLIOMYELITIS

The first large scale application of natural foods and improved nutrition was at the *Sister Elizabeth Kenny Hospital* for the Treatment of Poliomyelitis in El Monte, California, where Miss Kenny lived and worked for the last years of her professional life. She believed that *the poor nutritional state of American children—too much candy, soft drinks, cake and cookies, white bread, and sugar—made polio cases here much worse,* with more paralysis, than she had seen in Australia and England.

As Chief of Staff I persuaded Dr. Walsh to become the nutritional consultant for the Sister Kenny Hospital. Along with Sister Kenny he introduced diets and menus which eliminated the deficient foods, dramatically aiding the recovery of paralyzed children and adults.

Preliminary research on the nutrition of poliomyelitis patients showed that *paralysis developed more often in children with diets containing excessive refined carbohydrates.* It was also discovered that *poliomyelitis, a viral disease, responded to vitamin C therapy.* Massive doses of vitamin C helped control the acute stage and symptoms of polio and reduce the extent and severity of the paralysis. It appeared to be life-saving in 7 acutely ill patients with temperatures over 104° F. who were developing bulbar and spinal paralysis. Within 48 hours of vitamin C therapy, as much as 20 grams intravenously, the fevers subsided and they all went on to good recoveries.

When the Sister Kenny Hospital in El Monte closed we organized a crippled children's clinic and convalescent hospital in *Desert Hot Springs, California,* to treat the residual paralysis of some of our little patients and to carry on the diet and nutritional methods started at El Monte. Three public spiritied citizens—Leslie S. Morgan, C.C. Covey, and A.L. Eaton—founded the *Angel View Crippled Children Foundation* in a rented store building. The fees of adult patients treated in the morning paid the expenses of children treated free of charge in the afternoons. Along with nutritional therapy the children were exercised daily in the natural hot mineral water pools, a geological feature of that city.

When philanthropist Audrey Wardman came to our aid we soon had an out-patient clinic, our own hot mineral water therapeutic pool, and a 16-bed convalescent hospital wing. Here the children received natural foods, physical therapy, and medical care—and they recovered more rapidly than patients with similar conditions elsewhere in the United States. Eventually the hospital enlarged to 50 beds and became a custodial home for spastic children.

THE FIRST ARTHRITIS PATIENTS

As the number of poliomyelitis patients decreased we began to accept children with *Still's disease, a juvenile form of rheumatoid arthritis.* We found, first, that *hot mineral water baths and physical therapy would relieve the pain, swelling, and stiffness of their inflamed joints.* We included them in the nutritional therapy and special natural food menus given to the polio patients. The changes and improvement in these arthritic children were dramatic! We had made a second discovery that brought hope and healing to all patients with rheumatic diseases: *nutrional therapy helps cure arthritis!*

CASE HISTORY:

Alice was only five years old, but for two years she had suffered with multiple joint involvement from rheumatoid arthritis. Her hips and knees were so contracted she could only lie on her side; she could not sit in a chair. She was no larger than a small 3-year-old. Her joints were so painful when moved that she had to be carried into the hospital on a large pillow. For the previous two years she had been a patient in three well-known children's and orthopedic hospitals and had become progressively worse. Finally her parents were told to take her home, that there was not hope of any improvement or cure.

Considering the severity of her disease we very much

doubted if *any* treatment would improve her grave condition. But the "whole patient" approach was successful beyond *all* previous experience we had had with arthritis patients.

In our hospital Alice was given hours of special nursing care and nutritional attention. She was fed 5 small meals a day of fresh blended vegetable juices, natural fruit juices, eggs, and certified raw milk. She was given liquid vitamin supplements of cod liver oil, vitamin C, and vitamin B-complex in therapeutic doses and all her previous arthritis drugs were gradually withdrawn.

On warm days she lay in the sunshine until her milk white skin acquired a light tan. She was gently placed in the warm therapeutic pool three times a day for relief of pain and to improve circulation, and a therapist exercised each of her joints under the mineral waters.

Within 4 weeks the pain and swelling of her joints had subsided enough for her to sit in a chair. In three months she was standing and learning to swim. In six months she was discharged—by then she was walking and riding her tricycle. The tearful gratitude of her parents was one of the rare compensations of medical practice, making all the struggle of fighting disease and death worthwhile.

CASE HISTORY:

Johnny was seven years old and had been treated for Still's disease at a famous medical school hospital with the corticosteroid drugs. His face was swelled like a chubby little frog and he walked like a bow-legged cowboy, with stiff hips and feet well apart. His fingers were straight and stiff on swollen hands and wrists, and he could not dress or feed himself. On drug therapy, he was having no pain and gave us a wonderful smile. But in spite of the suppressive effect of the medication he had been slowly and steadily getting worse. He had developed the edema and pale skin of anemia. The drugs had been increased to the maximum he could tolerate.

Without making any promises, we accepted Johnny as an in-patient for the same treatment routine we had found successful with Alice. The aspirin and cortisone were decreased. At first he had more pain, irritability, and depression—although part of this may have been homesickness in his new surroundings. But he enjoyed the hot mineral pools and swimming exercises and became interested in the school and activity programs he shared with the other children.

Within a few weeks the swelling in his face and the edema in his hands and feet had disappeared. Within three months he was off all arthritic drugs. He was eating twice as much as he could tolerate on admission, including the certified raw milk. X-rays showed some permanent joint damage, which persisted in only one elbow and one ankle as he improved. His hips took three years to fully heal. Johnny was *the first patient we had ever seen to experience complete regeneration of new and normal bone in severe rheumatoid joints.*

When Angel View was closed for two years we opened the free *Desert Crippled Children Clinic* in Desert Hot Springs, where Alice and Johnny and over 300 other children have been examined and treated in the past 15 years. Alice is now a high school senior and a good swimmer. She has only some growth retardation to show for her previous disease. Johnny lives on a ranch in Colorado, rides horses, and has no real physical handicap from the residual stiffness in two of his limbs. Both children followed the nutritional program through all of their growing years and have been healthier than average children with fewer infections and less severe childhood illnesses.

THESE TWO PIONEER CASES began a series of patients with arthritis and other rheumatoid diseases who have been successfully treated by nutritional therapy and hot mineral baths at Desert Hot Springs, California, over the past 20 years. During this time we have learned much that is valuable in the dietary management of these conditions. Yet *much remains to be investigated and proven before such routines are accepted and used by the rest of the medical profession.*

Experimental arthritis is difficult to produce, and animals generally do not have arthritis, so studies in this field must be made on human subjects. It has been suggested that we prove our results by treating some patients with special diets and an equal number of "control" patients on regular diets, then compare the two groups. Although this may very well be done with animals, our patients are not guinea pigs. *Every patient is entitled to the best possible treatment and the latest discoveries,* regardless of whether or not nutritional therapy and the effect of natural hot mineral water baths have been confirmed by animal experiments or on human controls in a parallel series of experiments.

D. DIETARY AND HAIR ANALYSIS

DIETARY ANALYSIS

The most important information on diet is found in the medical history of the patient himself. The patient should compile a record of all food and drink consumed for a full week which is typical of his diet. This information is then statistically compared by a computer with "normal" standards—based on the patient's age, sex, weight, physical activity, and general health.

The final computer report reveals the food components in the patient's diet and the percentages of deficiencies or excesses in each vital food category.

The dietary analysis provides the following specific information:

WEIGHT. Whethet the patient is overweight or underweight, and whether this is related to an excessive or deficient intake of total calories.

NUTRIENTS. The patient's intake of nutritious foods (*proteins,* necessary *carbohydrates,* essential *fats*) and processed foods containing an excess of "empty" *calories* (white flour, white sugar) and hydrogenated oils, adding an excessively high fat content to the diet.

VITAMINS AND MINERALS. The patient's intake of *essential vitamins* and *minerals* (including calcium, phosphorus, iron, magnesium) and trace minerals (such as iodine, magnesium).

ACID/BASE RATIO. This ratio may be important in dental caries, pyorrhea and *osteoporosis.*

DIETARY ANALYSIS

The dietary analysis concludes with a computer printout of general information on diet and health according to the individual patient's needs and with discussions and recommendations for treatment. Prepared by authorities in human nutrition, it is written in terms that the average person can understand.

The dietary analysis has proven to be 95% accurate in revealing the patient's true nutritional status because most people follow the same food patterns week after week. The increased incidence of some types of arthritis in certain families, races, or geographical areas are more closely related to food patterns than to heredity or locality. Family habits, food preferences, allergies, and even racial and religious food patterns also influence the final dietary analysis of many patients.

Although every patient's dietary analysis is unique, the similarities of patients with the same types of arthritis are significant and often point to the origins of their diseases. But deficiencies vary greatly from patient to patient, and each must be considered separately, both in diagnosis and treatment.

Two common dietary factors are found in nearly every arthritis patient, regardless of diagnosis, and which may be the main contributing factors in the cause of all arthritis: *(1) an abnormally low intake of protein and (2) an abnormally high intake of refined carbohydrates.* Most arthritis patients have *not* followed a well-balanced diet conducive to good health. Serious dietary deficiencies and the intake of toxic or allergenic foods may contribute directly to their arthritis condition and may even be one of the causes of the disease.

VITAMIN THERAPY

Arthritis patients need more than the normal maintenance intake of protein, vitamins, and minerals. They are placed on a mega-vitamin therapy program— a double or triple supply of vitamins and food supplements—for three to six months, or until they appear to make maximum improvement from nutritional therapy. Then they may reduce their intake of therapeutic vitamins and minerals by at least one half. But they need to maintain a higher level of these food concentrates than the average person for the rest of their lives.

HAIR ANALYSIS

Trace element nutrition and metabolism play a significant role in the maintenance of health. New methods in clinical diagnosis allow the early assessment of metabolic trends.

Mineral excesses or deficiencies found in the hair may be related to some forms of arthritis. Substantial laboratory and clinical research support the analysis of hair as an ideal tissue source for the diagnosis of mineral trace element levels, for the following reasons:

1. Standard blood or urine tests are inadequate in indentifying chronic, subclinical effects from environmental exposure to potentially toxic elements such as lead, cadmium, mercury, and aluminum.

2. Serum levels of essential elements reflect extracellular levels and activity, providing a different and perhaps unrelated look at an instant in time. Endogenous hair trace element levels reflect the intracellular levels and total metabolic consequence of trace elements in the body over a period of time. And hair levels have been correlated with organ tissue levels.

3. Hair specimens are easy to obtain; collection is non-invasive and non-traumatic. Specimens are biologically stable and will not deteriorate in transit.

COLLECTING AND HANDLING HAIR SPECIMENS

QUANTITY. Because of variations in growth cycle and other factors, contiguous hairs on the scalp can have reasonably varied trace element concentrations. Only a sufficient sample (hundreds of hairs) will yield a significant average value. One gram of hair provides the ideal sample size.

LENGTH. Hair grows about half an inch per month. The most recent period of growth (two to four months) is preferred so the sample should be no longer than one and one half to two inches from the scalp. Longer hair lengths pick up considerably more exogenous contaminants, presumably from its unwinding which results in greater porosity of the hair protein.

LOCATION. The suboccipital region of the head provides the most consistent specimen, even for those who are balding.

CONDITION. Cold waving and bleaching can cause significant alterations in the mineral content of hair and produce poor specimens for tissue mineral analysis. Other hair treatments do not seem to affect mineral content significantly except for shampoos containing high levels of zinc or selenium and progressive hair dyes containing lead. However, these effects are easily recognized and do not interfere with the accurate reflection of other hair minerals.

Qualified laboratories report the findings of diet and hair analyses in about seven to ten days after submissions by the referring physicians.

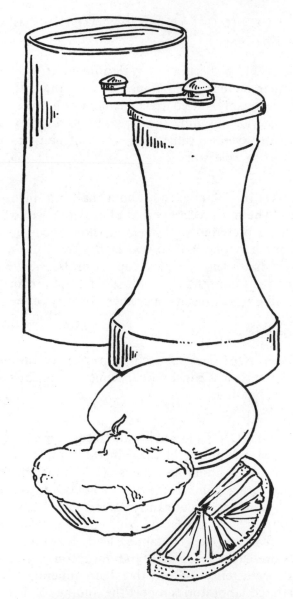

**SEASONINGS AND HERBS
ARE RICH IN VITAMINS**

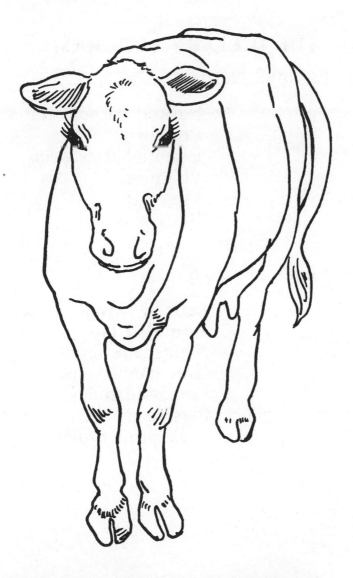

MILK IS MAN'S, AND WOMAN'S,
BEST FOOD FOR ARTHRITIS
PREVENTION AND TREATMENT

Table 10
THE DIETARY PROGRAM
1. Essential Nutrients

Natural carbohydrates
Protein
Essential fatty acids
Vitamins
Minerals
Fiber

2. Foods to Avoid

Refined carbohydrates
Saturated fats
Nightshade foods
Over cooked meals
Processed foods
Preserved foods
High protein diets

CHAPTER 10

THE DIETARY PROGRAM

Like plants, our bodies need lime, potash, phosphate, manganese, and zinc. But they also require many chemicals that green plants can make for themselves—valine, leucine, phenylalanine, and tryptophan—as well as an undetermined number of vitamins and other nutrients.

Just as the health and vigor of a plant depends on a good supply of the required chemicals, *the health and vitality of the human body depends on the external supply of essential body chemicals.*

Nutritional science teaches us (1) how crucial the internal environment of our body cells and tissues is; (2) that the nutrition we receive in food may shape and build our entire lives; and (3) that all kinds of diseases and malformations are rooted in poor internal environment from dietary deficiencies.

Nutrients, (vitamins, food supplments, etc.) should *not* be considered as *medicinal agents,* as they function in an entirely different way. Medicines and drugs interfere with metabolism, but nutrients make metabolism possible. They are the raw materials from which metabolic machinery is built and life cannot exist without them.

The intricate balance of nutrients in the body involves the inter-relationships among forty or more such substances. *An extremely poor nutritional balance may result in deficiency diseases;* a poor or mediocre balance yields at best sub-optimal health and vigor.

A balanced diet in the ordinary sense does not guard against developmental errors or nutrition-related disease, the origins of which are as obscure as our knowledge of nutrition is limited. A large percentage of Americans eat the customary foods and yet have a poor or mediocre internal environment.

Adjusting internal environments to avoid disease cannot be done in terms of lettuce, beefsteak, and beans. But the nutrient minerals, amino acids, and vitamins of these foods reach the body's cells and tissues and are essential to their life.

"Body wisdom" is an instinct that prevents an individual from eating a pound of butter, sugar, or salt even though the first taste may be tempting. It is not the same in all individuals. Since animals can differentiate between balanced and unbalanced nutrients in their selection of foods, so also can humans. But how it can be cultivated and implemented is largely unexplored territory.

Nutrition has been in lethargy for too long. It needs to be taken seriously by biochemists, medical scientists, medical educators, and family physicians. Vast human betterment—including substantial relief from coronary heart disease, birth defects, arthritis, mental disease, alcoholism, dental disease, muscular dystrophy, mulitple sclerosis, cataracts, glaucoma, cancer, and many other diseases—must await the day when nutrition comes alive and reaches out to new horizons.

A. THE ESSENTIAL NUTRIENTS

The body requires protein, carbohydrates, essential fats, fiber, vitamins and minerals for its proper function and optimum health. All these nutrients must be obtained in the proper proportions or the rest cannot work effectively, and mental or physical impairment or disease will result.

A sound foundation of the basic essential nutrients should be established first; then the individual should concentrate on food sources rich in specific nutrients as required by illness or deficiency. The harmful effects of pollutants and environmental poisons require extra protection, such as the antioxidant properties of vitamins E, C, and A. *Extra B vitamins and vitamin C are required to help the body cope with stress.*

Much of our produce today is grown for size or quantity rather than quality, treated with chemical fertilizers and pesticides, harvested before it is ripe, transported long distances, stored for long periods, and finally processed and packaged. By the time it reaches the consumer, much of its food value has been lost or destroyed.

Processing destroys many valuable nutrients— especially vitamins and enzymes—through sterilization and overheating. Over-refining removes many valuable trace minerals found in the outer casing of grains. Food additives in packaged foods may introduce undesirable and even harmful chemicals to the diet.

Consequently, foods that are raw, fresh, and naturally grown are far more nutritious and healthful than processed or refined foods. Vitamins can be replaced by daily food supplements, *but many enzymes are available only in fresh milk, fruit and vegetables.* Frozen foods have lost some of their food value but are much preferred over canned and packaged foods.

Care must also be taken in the home preparation of food to retain valuable nutrients. *Overcooking and too-high temperatures are probably the most common problems—destroying some vitamins and removing enzymes and trace minerals into the cooking water.* Rancidity, however slight, destroys many nutrients and can also produce reactions in some sensitive and allergic people. Oils, salad dressings, butter, peanut butter, etc. should be refrigerated; coffee should not be reheated.

PROTEIN

Protein is the first essential nutrient of life and is imperative in maintaining good health. Since it provides amino-acids and nitrogen for building body tissue, it is necessary for growth and devlopment; it can also be used as an energy source if necessary.

The most important components of dietary protein are the eight amino acids (plus histidine for infants). *These cannot be produced by the body but must be supplied in the diet.* All essential amino acids must be present together in the digestive tract at the same time in order to be properly utilized by the body. If even one is missing or ingested several hours later, body protein cannot be produced and they will be used for energy instead. Excess protein, not used for building tissue or for energy, is converted to fat and stored in the body tissues and cannot be converted back to protein.

Complete protein foods contain all the essential amino acids and these include most dairy products and meats. *Incomplete protein* foods are low and lacking in an essential amino acid and they include most grains, nuts, and vegetables. An incomplete protein food, however, can become "complete" when combined with a food containing the missing amino acid.

CARBOHYDRATES

Carbohydrates provide the major energy source for metabolic functions, physical activity, and growth. They also aid in digestion and regulate protein and fat metabolism.

Carbohydrates enter the body mainly as sugars and starches found in whole grains, legumes, fresh fruits and vegetables. These *natural, unrefined carbohydrates provide many important vitamins and minerals as well as the necessary bulk for a healthy digestive system.* Refined carbohydrates are not only "fattening" but may contribute to the development of heart disease, diabetes, high blood pressure, and dental caries as well as poor appetite and food habits, fuzzy vision, dizziness, and a generally "rotten" feeling. They also retard the growth of valuable intestinal bacteria and encourage fermentation and gas in the gastrointestinal tract. Refined carbohydrates should be eliminated entirely, if possible, as the refining process has removed most of the trace elements necessary for the metabolism of sugars in the body.

Refined sugar is found in candy, soft drinks, and prepared desserts as well as "hidden" in many packaged and prepared foods. Cooked desserts made with honey are partially refined since much of the food value has been destroyed by heating, leaving mostly sugar.

About 55-65% of the body's caloric intake should come from natural carbohydrates. Carbohydrate deficiencies prevent the body from getting full value from the available protein and would hinder the breaking down of fats. Protein destruction and acidosis result when proteins are burned for energy rather than utilized for body building.

Natural starches are slowly converted by the body into sugar, giving a steady supply of energy. But refined sugars and refined starches—such as processed white flour, white rice, potato chips, and alcohol—are quickly converted into sugar and dumped into the system, overstimulating the production of insulin and digestive juice.

FATS

Body fats form a protective cover over the delicate internal organs and play an important role in metabolism by releasing certain chemical substances (such as cholesterol, triglycerides, free fatty acids) for use by the body.

However, blood *lipid (fat) abnormalities are related to heart and vascular disease, and excessive fat intake has been linked to cancer, obesity, premature aging, and indigestion.* The typical American diet has an intake of over 40% calories from fat, whereas a level of 10-30% is usually considered optimum. Besides butter, oils and mayonnaise many "hidden" sources contribute to the excessive consumption of fats: gravies, sauces, nuts, pastries, whole dairy products, and fatty meats.

The role of dietary fat is not yet fully understood, but during digestion it is broken down into fatty acids. The three essential ones—*linoleic, linolenic, and arachidonic acid—cannot be produced by the body and are necessary for normal healthy skin, arteries, blood, glands, and nerves* as well as for breaking down cholesterol and saturated fats.

Unrefined oils provide *vitamin E* and the essential fatty acids. The best sources are natural, "unsaturated" ("non-hydrogenated," "polyunsaturated") nuts, grains, and liquid fish and vegetable oils. Safflower (linoleic), soy (linolenic), and peanut (arachindonic) oils are highest in essential fatty acids; Other good sources are sunflower and sesame seeds, walnuts, corn, and cottonseed; of lesser value are avocados, other nuts and nut butters, some mayonnaises, and olive oil. *Consumption of "saturated" ("hardened," "solid," "hydrogenated") fats should be limited,* especially in the absence of sufficient essential fatty acids for breaking them down in the body. These animal and milk fats are excessively supplied in dairy products and meats such as pork and fatty beef. "Hardened" oils are found in many frozen and prepared bakery products, some nut butters, potato chips, and restaurant-prepared fried foods. Many packaged foods are prepared with unspecified "vegetable oils."

Essential fatty acids can be destroyed by processing (hydrogenation), frying, and exposure to heat, light, or air. Therefore it is important to store nuts and other fat or oil containing foods in dark, covered containers away from direct light and under refrigeration to prevent rancidity. Avoid heating such foods whenever posssible.

DIETARY FIBER

Dietary fiber includes plant components not digested in the small intestine such as cellulose, hemicellulose, lignin, pectin, etc. Each has different properties and appears in varying composition in plants. To obtain the maximum benefit from the different properties of dietary fiber, *it is advisable to select a variety of high-fiber foods rather than rely on only one or two sources.*

Insufficient dietary fiber has been associated with atherosclerosis, diabetes, heart disease, diverticulitis, constipation, varicose veins, hiatus hernia, appendicitus, and hemorrhoids. Natural dietary fibers found in whole grains, nuts, legumes, fruits, and vegetables are often low from over-refining and processing, which depletes much of their fiber content.

Products that contain "non-nutritive fiber" should be avoided, as some may contain wood pulp or sawdust to increase fiber content.

ACID/BASE RATIO (ASH)

Foods burned by the body leave a residue, or ash, which is either acid, alkaline, or neutral depending on the mineral content of the food. *A healthy digestive system and a normally functioning liver will maintain a proper acid/alkaline balance through a buffering system.* A disturbance in the balance, however, will result in acidosis or alkalosis of the blood and can be prevented to some degree by proper diet. Alkaline ash is produced by vegetables and most fruits (except cranberries, plums, and prunes). Acidic ash is produced by most proteins and grain foods. Butter, oils, honey, and milk are considered neutral.

B. THE MAIN FOOD GROUPS

MEATS

Liver and other organ meats are excellent sources of protein, the B vitamins and other vitamins, iron, and trace minerals. Fresh lamb, pork, chicken, or calves' liver should be eaten once a week, preferably at breakfast. *Lean beef or lamb, poultry, fish, and seafood supply protein, iron, and phosphorus; in addition, seafood and ocean fish furnish iodine and trace minerals.*

Serve meat daily unless sufficient proteins are supplied from other sources such as eggs, milk, cheese, and liver. Visible fat should be removed, and be careful not to overcook. Choose fresh or frozen meats rather than canned (except for tuna and salmon). Pork, ham, and bacon—which are high in fats and must be well-cooked—should be eaten sparingly, if at all; processed or packaged meats (such as hot dogs, lunchmeats, salami) contain much fat and chemicals and should be avoided entirely.

FRUITS AND VEGETABLES

Fresh, naturally grown fruits and vegetables are superior in food value to frozen or canned produce—especially when eaten raw. They supply potassium and a small amount of minerals and vitamins. If cooked, they should be heated only until tender, using little or no water.

Dark green or yellow vegetables and fruits (leafy greens, carrots, squash, sweet potato, asparagus, apricots, peaches) are rich in vitamin A, folic acid, and magnesium. Citrus fruits and fresh juices with pulp (such as orange and grapefruit), papaya, cantalope, strawberries, broccoli, and sweet pepper contain vitamin C. Naturally ripened or sun-dried fruits provide potassium, natural sugar, carotene, vitamin C, and several trace minerals.

GRAINS AND NUTS

Fresh, stoneground cereals, corn meal, and flour supply B vitamins, iron, some protein, vitamin E, and minerals. But *bread is the "staff of life" only when it is made from the whole grain and contains the vitamins and trace minerals found in the germ, or berry, of the grain.* Therefore, choose only *wholegrain* products: brown rice, whole wheat and rye, yellow corn meal, buckwheat, millet, oats, freshly milled wheat germ.

Natural whole grain rice is a good substitute for bread when allergies or gastrointestinal conditions are present. It is also a good source for carbohydrates and calories in growing children. *Wheat germ (freshly milled) or bran may be added to other cereals, pancakes, waffles, muffins, etc.* Granola is the best cold cereal.

Nuts and seeds should be whole, fresh, and unsalted

(sunflower, pumpkin, and sesame seeds, almonds, walnuts, etc.). Nut butters should be non-hydrogenated and without additives; to obtain a lower fat content, pour off excess oil from the top. Avoid cracked nuts or broken pieces, which are often rancid.

Avoid foods made from enriched, refined flours (refined pastas; bakery products and prepared mixes; packaged cereals, cookies, cakes, and pastries; "enriched" white breads, cereals, and crackers). About 20 nutrients are refined out of white flour.

MILK

Milk is the first food of infancy and the last of old age. Cow's or goat's milk and their products should be served at every meal. *Two or 3 glasses a day (or the equivalent in dairy products such as buttermilk, cottage cheese, and yogurt) provide most of the essential vitamins and trace minerals our bodies need.*

Fresh milk from the dairy is richer in vitamin C than carton milk from the market. *Certified raw milk* if available, *is highly recommended.* It is higher in enzymes, hormone growth factors, Wulzen factor, protein, available minerals and fats, and natural vitamins than pasteurized milk. It is especially valuable for those with a tendency to arthritis and for underdeveloped children. Skim milk has had most of the cream and butterfat removed, along with most of the trace minerals (yet these minerals are required for the proper digestion and utilization of the skim milk). *Buttermilk has the same protein value as whole milk and contains no more fat than skim milk.*

Besides as a beverage, milk may be used in custards, cream soups, gravies and sauces. Yogurt, one of the principal food sources in countries where people regularly live to more than 100 years of age, goes well with fruit and in salads, and is essential in high protein and low fat reducing diets. Cottage cheese is a good base for fruit and vegetable salads.

Eggs may be substituted for most meats, providing the daily protein requirement along with iron, vitamin A, and especially methionine. Choose fertile eggs when possible.

Natural, *unprocessed cheeses* (Jack, Gouda, etc.) are an excellent source of protein and far more nutritious than processed, chemicalized cheeses, spreads, and margarines (American, cream cheese, etc.). Skim milk cheese is a suitable alternative. Cheeses may be used in a wide variety of dishes—omelets, souffles, fondues, blintzes, rarebit, or as toppings for vegetables.

C. RAW VS. PASTEURIZED MILK

1. FACILITY TESTING AND INSPECTIONS

MILK

Certified raw milk is available only in a few favored areas of this country. It is tested daily for bacteria at an independent laboratory for the Certified Milk Commission. *The standard plate count (total of all bacteria in the milk) may not exceed 10,000/ml* of raw milk and cream; the coliform (normally foreign) bacterial count is limited to a maximum of 10/ml. Streptococci tests are made monthly, and the brucella ring test is performed at least 4 times a year; if positive, the entire herd is blood tested and any positive reactors are removed.

Pasteurized milk is tested monthly for bacteria by the County Health Department. The standard plate count before pasteurization may not exceed **50,000/ml** of raw milk; *after pasteurization, the maximum is*

15,000/ml of milk and 25,000/ml of cream. The coliform bacterial count is limited to 750/ml of raw milk and 10/ml of pasteurized milk. The brucella ring test is also conducted at least 4 times a year.

DAIRY HERD

All dairy cows in a certified milking herd are inspeced at least weekly by a herd sanitarian from the County Medical Milk Commission and monthly by a County Health Inspector. All cows are blood tested for brucellosis when first entering the herd, and annually thereafter (any positive reactors are removed). Those between 2 and 6 months old are vaccinated for brucellosis. A skin test for tuberculosis is performed annually by a state veterinarian and any positive reactors are removed.

Salmonella bacteria have been a cause for concern by the health department. They are occasionally found in raw milk. However there is no proven case of illness from salmonella from raw certified milk.

All cows at a pasteurized milk dairy are inspected monthly by a County Health Inspector. The brucellosis vaccination and TB skin test are the same as for certified herds. However, the brucellosis blood test is performed only on those cows imported into California.

DAIRY EMPLOYEES

All employees at a certified dairy undergo a complete physical examination upon hiring, and monthly examinations are conducted thereafter. In addition, a streptococcus throat culture and examination is made monthly; a stool specimen is taken twice a year; and a TB chest x-ray or skin test is given annually.

Employees at a pasteurized milk dairy are given physical examination only upon hiring. No regular examinations are given thereafter.

2. NUTRITIONAL VALUES

ENZYMES

Enzymes are unstable, organic substances that act as metabolic catalysts and are required for digestion. They are easily destroyed or inactivated by high temperatures or a wide variety of chemical substances. *The enzymes catalase, peroxidase, and phosphatase are all present in raw milk;* but *pasteurization destroys the enzyme phosphatase, which is required to split and assimilate mineral salts in foods that are in the form of phytates.*

GROWTH FACTORS

The Wulzen Factor (anti-stiffness) is available in raw milk. Test animals on raw milk show normal growth and no abnormalities. This factor is destroyed in pasteurization; test animals on processed milk do not grow well and develop a definite syndrome, beginning with wrist stiffness.

The X Factor (tissue repair) available in raw milk is also present in pasteurized milk with no evidence of alteration.

PROTEIN

All 22 amino acids, including the 8 essential for complete metabolism and the function of protein, are 100% metabolically available in raw milk. After pasteurization, however, digestibility is reduced by 4% and biological value is reduced by 17%. Digestibility and metabolic data indicate that heat destroys the identity of lysine (and possibly histidine and other amino acids) and partly decreases the absorbability of their nitrogen.

World-wide population studies seem to indicate that the large increase of heart disease in the Western world is correlated with the onset of pasteurization and may be due to the fact that the heat process of pasteurization alters the protein found in raw milk.

VITAMINS

Of all the vitamins, 100% available in raw milk, only vitamins D, E, and K are unaltered by pasteurization. Vitamin A and the antineuretic vitamin are destroyed completely, and about 38% of the B-complex vitamins are destroyed by pasteurization (infants fed pasteurized milk exclusively may develop scurvy).

MINERALS

The 7 major minerals (calcium, chlorine, magnesium, phosphorus, potassium, sodium, sulphur) and all 24 (or more) vital trace minerals are 100% metabolically available in raw milk. *But pasteurization diminishes the total soluble calcium available,* which is an important factor in the growth and development of infants and children (in the formation of bone and teeth as well as the calcium content of the blood).

CARBOHYDRATES

Carbohydrates easily utilized in metabolism remain associated naturally with elements in raw milk, with no evidence of alteration by pasteurization.

FATS

All 18 fatty acids, both saturated and unsaturated, are metabolically available in raw milk. Pasteurization alters and harms the fat content of milk by reducing the size of the fat particles and permitting them to be assimilated into the stomach lining in a manner not intended by nature. Along with xanthine oxidase, these fat particles get into the blood stream and trigger the body's defense mechanism, resulting in the eventual scarring of arteries and arteriosclerosis.

Homogenization reduces the size of the fat elements in milk and may be another factor in the causes of hardening of the arteries.

C. RECOMMENDED MENUS

The following 2-week menu schedule is based on a nutrition program that eliminates the "nightshade" plants and includes many items to enrich the nutrition of each meal.

Although they are not nightshade products, *coffee and tea are not recommended beverages* with these menus. Excessive consumption may cause facial rash or chest pains. Decaffeinated coffee may be substituted, but do not sweeten. Soft drinks should be avoided because of their sugar, caffeine, and fluoride content. Alcohol should be restricted because of the damage it does to tissues.

Sunday

Breakfast
Stewed Apples
Granola with Milk
or
Buckwheat Pancakes with Butter &
Honey
Orange Juice

Lunch
Cranberry Juice
Baked Lamb or Sea Slaw
Corn-on-the-Cob
Steamed Broccoli
Fresh Pineapple
Beverage

Dinner
Turkey Loaf
Raw Vegetable Salad
Steamed Cauliflower with Cheese Sauce
Whole Grain Bread and Butter
Raw Fruit
Beverage

Monday

Breakfast
Orange Juice
Granola with Milk
or
Soft Cooked Egg
Rye Toast and Butter
Beverage

Lunch
Banana Squash Soup
Baked Veal
Raw Carrot Curls
Celery and Watercress Salad
Yogurt and Sliced Banana
Beverage

Dinner
Chicken Salad
Steamed Carrots and Green Peas
Whole Grain Bread and Butter
Wedge of Melon (in season)
Beverage

Tuesday

Breakfast
Cranberry Juice
Malt-O-Meal with Milk
or
Poached Egg
Whole Grain Bread and Butter
Beverage

Lunch
Chicken-Rice Casserole
Green Beans O'Brien
Fresh Fruit Salad
Rye Bread and Butter
Beverage

Dinner
Baked Fish with Lemon Sauce
Zucchini with Mushrooms
Raw Applesauce
Tossed Green Salad
Beverage

Wednesday

Breakfast
Stewed Prunes
Granola with Milk
or
Buckwheat Pancakes with Honey Butter
Beverage

Lunch
Boiled Beef Brisket
Oven-browned Turnips
Fresh Fruit Salad with Cheese
Baked Yams
Whole Wheat Bread and Butter
Beverage

Dinner
Chicken-bone Vegetable Soup
Calf Liver with Onion Rings
Vegetable-egg Salad
or
Carrot and Celery Salad
Beverage

Thursday

Breakfast
Half Grapefruit
Ralston with Milk
or
Hard Cooked Egg
Cracked Wheat Bread and Butter
Beverage

Lunch
Salisbury Steak
Lemon-buttered Spinach
Orange-apple Salad
or
Yogurt and Fresh Fruit
Rye Bread and Butter
Beverage

Dinner
Vegetable Broth
Macaroni and Cheese
Fresh Sliced Apple
or
Rye Bread and Butter
Beverage

Friday

Breakfast
Banana
Granola and Milk
or
Beef Patty
Rye Bread and Butter
Beverage

Lunch
Salmon Patty with Egg Sauce
Carrots and Peas
Sliced Beet Salad
or
Steamed Brown Rice
Fresh Pear with Cheese
Beverage

Dinner
Beef and Scalloped Corn Casserole
Peas and Carrots
Fresh Grapes and Cheese
or
Yogurt and Fresh Fruit
Beverage

Saturday

Breakfast
Stewed Prunes
Ralston with Milk
or
Hard Cooked Egg
Cracked Wheat Bread and Butter
Beverage

Lunch
Lentil Soup
Broiled Fillet Steak
Peas and Button Mushrooms
Vegetable Salad
Apple Pudding
Beverage

Dinner
Vegetable Soup
Cottage Cheese and Fresh Pear Salad
Steamed Green Beans
Beverage

Sunday

Breakfast
Orange Slices
Malt-O-Meal
or
Poached Eggs
Rye Bread and Butter
Beverage

Lunch
Celery Soup with Mushrooms
Swiss Steak with Noodles and Gravy
Raw Cabbage Salad
Beverage

Dinner
Chicken-Rice Casserole
Green Bean and Red Onion Salad
or
Fresh Fruit Salad
Whole Grain Bread and Butter
Beverage

Monday

Breakfast
Grape Juice
Oatmeal with Fresh Fruit and Milk
or
French Toast with Honey Butter
Beverage

Lunch
Carrot Soup
Chicken or Lamb Meat Loaf
Honey-glazed Banana Squash
or
Cauliflower with Cheese Sauce
Fresh Pineapple
Beverage

Dinner
Roast Lamb and Gravy
Escalloped Squash
Tossed Green Salad
or
Stewed Mixed Dried Fruit
Whole Grain Bread and Butter
Beverage

Tuesday

Breakfast
Carrot Juice
Granola with Milk and Grated Apple
or
Soft Cooked Egg
Bran Muffin or Corn Bread and Butter
Beverage

Lunch
Baked Chicken-Noodle Casserole
Brussel Sprouts and Steamed Beets
or
Green Bean Salad
Fresh Pear with Cheese Wedge
Beverage

Dinner
Split Pea Soup
Cottage Cheese and Fresh Fruit
Whole Grain Bread and Peanut Butter
Beverage

Wednesday

Breakfast
Baked Apple with Yogurt
Oatmeal with Milk
or
French Toast with Orange Butter
Beverage

Lunch
Green Pea Soup
Roast Chicken
Baked Sweet Potato
Grapes and Banana Salad
Whole Grain Bread and Butter
Beverage

Dinner
Eggs Goldenrod
Green Peas and Onions
Carrot, Raisin and Celery Salad
or
Tangerine with Cheese Wedge
Whole Wheat Bread and Butter
Beverage

Thursday

Breakfast
Sliced Orange
Oatmeal with Milk
or
Poached Eggs
Whole Grain Bread and Butter
Beverage

Lunch
Baked Fish
Green Beans
Fresh Fruit Salad
Yogurt and Fresh Fruit
Beverage

Dinner
Sloppy Joe on Whole Grain Bun
Corn Niblets
Broccoli Spears with Mushroom Sauce
or
Yogurt and Fresh Vegetable Salad
Rye Bread and Butter
Beverage

Friday

Breakfast
Half Grapefruit
Buckwheat Pancakes with Honey Butter
Beverage

Lunch
Vegetable Broth
Veal Steak with Mushroom Sauce
Spinach Souffle or Creamed Spinach
or
Fruit Salad with Cottage Cheese
and Yogurt Whip
Whole Grain Bread and Butter
Beverage

Dinner
Beef Patty on Rye Bread
Onion Rings
Cole Slaw
Carrot and Pineapple Salad
Beverage

CHAPTER 11

VITAMIN AND MINERAL THERAPY

ONE OF THE MOST POPULAR MEDICAL MYTHS is "All the nutrition you need for arthritis is a well balanced diet". This is far from the truth. First, well nourished persons seldom, if ever, come down with rheumatic diseases. Second, because of the reduced capacity for physical exertion, inability to do heavy work or extensive exercise, their food consumption is diminished. Instead of "three square meals a day" the usual patient with arthritis problems may take less than half of that. If they exceed this limit they gain useless and handicapping weight for their painful joints to support. Such fat makes the patient's situation worse by increased fatigue of their affected limbs and impaired circulation to the spine and extremities.

The arthritic, then, from the beginnning of the disease is deficient in food, particularly proteins and essential fatty acids, but their meals are low in vitamins and minerals.

Dietary therapy, as applied to patients with all forms of arthritis, must therefore include those essential factors—the food catalysts which are necessary for body metabolism - vitamins, and the chemical building blocks which are contained in all cells and the blood - important minerals, such as calcium, iron and phosphorus, and trace minerals such as potassium, zinc, and magnesium, to name but a few.

A decline in food quality, a lack of natural foods, fresh fruit and vegetables, dairy products and whole grain cereals will contribute to inadequate vitamin and mineral intakes. An abundance of processed, preserved and "convenience foods", which lose much of their vitamin content during preparation and storage, can be an additional deterrent to good nutrition.

A. THERAPEUTIC VITAMINS.

VITAMIN D. This vitamin can be partially supplied by the exposure of skin to the sun. Removing the natural oils of the skin by too frequent washing with soap or skin detergents can reduce this beneficial energy. Persons whose activity limits their exposure to sunlight, and all arthritics, should obtain a dietary source of vitamin D, or regularly take a food supplement. Skin synthesis of this vitamin is limited by clouds, fog, smog and clothing by obstructing the sun's unltra-violet rays.

Natural sources of vitamin D-3, the food element, are eggs, liver, butter, sardines, salmon and fish liver oils. Synthetic vitamin D-2 is added to some homogenized milk, but organic origins are preferred.

Deficiencies in Vitamin D may lead to osteoarthritis, osteoporosis, malformed bones and poor teeth in children. It is essential for calcium and phosphorus metabolism and parathyroid imbalance. Minor symptoms include "growing pains" in youth, muscle cramps and constipation in adults.

The B COMPLEX vitamins and FOLIC ACID are the most common vitamin deficiencies. This can result from an inadequate intake, impaired absorption, excess stress or metabolic derangement. Infants, lactating women, adolescents and those with anemia, infections, and rheumatoid arthritis have increased requirements. Natural sources are wheat germ, brewer's yeast, green leafy vegetable, liver asparagus, lima beans and whole grain foods.

VITAMIN C is not only an essential vitamin for good health, but larger than minimum daily requirements is an important part of arthritis treatment. A lack of this factor may cause scurvy, but sub-clinical deficiencies contribute to frequent illnesses and infections, all forms of bone and joint disease, anemia, arteriosclerosis and heart disease. Recent studies suggest that larger than minimal amounts may protect against cancer. Body levels of vitamin C are decreased by such stresses as worry, fear, depression, excitement, fatigue, and by exposure to toxic metals, smog, chemicals and tobacco smoke.

Foods rich in vitamin C should be eaten every day, fresh and raw fruits and vegetables, fresh milk, berries, citrus fruit, broccoli, red cabbage, papaya and fruit juices.

LACK OF VITAMIN E is related to the poor circulation of arthritis patients. Treatment with this vitamin lessens fatigue, coldness in the extremities and may prevent heart disease, hardening of the arteries, strokes and premature physical degeneration, or "early aging." Taking mineral oil, frequent laxative, inorganic iron supplements, or rancid fats interfere with vitamin E absorption.

Foods rich in vitamin E are whole grains, corn, soy and safflower oil, raw nuts and seeds, soybeans and avocadoes. But for treatment purposes vitamin supplements of wheat germ oil are essential over a period of many months.

B. BASIC MINERALS

IRON DEFICIENCY is public health problem as well as an arthritis problem. It is one of the signs of rheumatoid disease and is frequent in infectious arthritis and osteoporosis. A lack of acid in the gastric juices, antacids, alcohol and coffee may interfere with absorption. Good iron sources are lean meats, liver, eggs, molasses, nuts and seed, leafy green, raisins, dates, oysters and clams. Taking vitamin C, ascorbic acid, in the same meal can enhance the digestion of iron rich foods.

IONIC OR DISSOLVED CALCIUM is one of the most important factors required for the proper function of the nervous and muscle systems and the building and repair of bone and cartilage. It is ionized through digestion and the action of vitamin D. A lack of calcium is signalled by spontaneous cramping of the muscles of the legs at night, layering and splitting of thin fingernails, and tenderness in the muscles. Demineralization of the skeleton may be seen in rheumatoid and osteoarthritis with osteoporosis, and may pre-date the appearance of clinical symptoms in many patients. Soft bone at the edges of the joints become "irritated" and cannot tolerate pressures, and "spurs" and "exostoses" are formed like little lips on the joint margins, a very characteristic finding in the x-rays of arthritis patients.

Dietary calcium is present in all dairy foods, meats, nuts and grains. Fish is deficient in calcium, which accounts for the small stature of Oriental peoples in the Far East, whose children and granchildren in this country grow taller and larger than their parents when raised on Western foods.

Calcium phosphate, calcium carbonate and calcium lactate can be taken as food supplements when the dietary supply has been inadequate for a long period of time. Protein-linked calcium orotate is effective in smaller dosage.

CALCIUM IS PRESENT in dairy products: milk, cheese, cream, egg yolk; vegetables: chard, cauliflower, kale, beans, rhubarb, beets, carrots, cabbage and spinach; fruits: dates, figs, lemons, oranges, pineapples, raspberries; seeds and grains: almonds, walnuts, bran and oatmeal; seafood: oysters and shell fish.

C. TRACE MINERALS

ZINC is a trace mineral, but the second most abundant mineral in the body. It is essential for wound healing and the repair of tissues damages by arthritis. The richest dietary origins are the high protein foods— whole grains, pumpkins seeds, oysters and yeast. Deficiencies are corrected by supplements, of zinc orotate after surgical operations, and by vitamin and mineral combinations in treating arthritis patients.

CHROMIUM IS NECESSARY for energy, strength and glucose metabolism. Inadequate amounts are related to diabetes, hypoglycemia, arteriosclerosis and hypertension. It is naturally found in brewer's yeast, liver, whole grains breads, mushrooms and beets. Multiple mineral supplements contain chromium.

COPPER is seldom lacking due to the common use of copper in water pipes for drinking water in most homes. An excess is more to be avoided than low levels, although a normal intake and tissue content is necessary in the treatment of rheumatoid arthritis. This may account for the popularity of "copper bracelets", which, while there is no scientific proof of their effectiveness, they certainly can do no harm.

Excessive copper may contribute to hyperactivity, insomnia, and hypertension; a lack may aggravate anemia. Small amounts are usually included in trace mineral combinations.

LEAD, ALUMINUM AND MERCURY ARE TOXIC MINERALS. Some physicians may not agree on the values of HAIR ANALYSIS in determining their presence in excessive amounts in the body. However, in our experience, where the hair analyses have shown these elements to be high in arthritis patients, reducing them to more acceptable levels has paralleled improvement in health.

THE "ONE A DAY" VITAMIN AND MINERAL SUPPLEMENTS are intended to compensate for the deficiencies in the daily diet from a decline in food quality, low intake and the stress of daily living. Patients with arthritis need more that these "minimum daily requirements", to build up their depleted reserves, to repair the bones and joints, and to FIGHT BACK AGAINST ARTHRITIS. For these reasons "therapeutic vitamins and minerals" are recommended, plus additional vitamin B complex, C, D, and E. After a dietary and hair analysis specific factors needed by the individual patient may be prescribed.

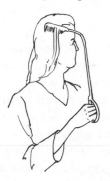

Table 11

VITAMIN AND MINERAL THERAPY

		DAILY MEGAVITAMIN THERAPY	DAILY MAINTENANCE
1. Essential Vitamins:	A	20,000 I.U.	10,000 I.U.
	B Complex	2 high potency tablets	1 tablet
	C	2,000 mg.	1,000 mg.
	D	800 I.U.	400 I.U.
	E	800 I.U.	400 I.U.
	Niacinamide	200 mg.	100 mg.
2. Essential Minerals:	Calcium	1,500 mg.	750 mg.
	Magnesium	750 mg.	375 mg.
3. Trace Minerals:	Iron	20 mg.	10 mg.
	Iodine	200 mg.	100 mg.
4. Optional Vitamins:	B 6	200 mg.	10 mg.
	Folic acid	400 mg.	20 mg.
	Biotin	200 mg.	10 mg.
	d-Calcium Pantothenate	20 mg.	10 mg.
5. Optional Minerals:	Copper	2 mg.	1 mg.
	Manganese	1 mg.	1 mg.
	Zinc	15 mg.	5 mg.
	Chromium	2 mg.	1 mg.

Table 12

YUCCA PLANT EXTRACT

CONSTITUENTS   Steroid Saponin

PROPERTIES   Improves blood circulation
Lowers blood cholesterol
   (When abnormal)
Lowers blood triglycerides
   (When abnormal)
Lowers blood pressure
   (When abnormal)

DOSAGE   300 mg. of Yucca Plant
Extract daily

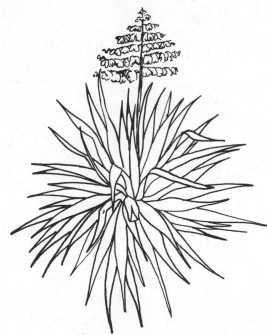

YUCCA IS A TRADITIONAL AMERICAN INDIAN REMEDY

CHAPTER 12

YUCCA PLANT EXTRACT

We have known for several years that a food *supplement extracted from yucca acts like a natural form of cortisone,* to reduce and eliminate the pain, swelling, and joint stiffness suffered by arthritis victims, with no side effects. There is also indisputable evidence that *this natural, non-toxic plant substance may prevent and correct several disorders originating in the gastrointestinal tract*—particularly *high blood pressure and excessive cholesterol and trilyceride levels in the blood.* We seem only to have scratched the surface of the medical uses of yucca.

A. HISTORY OF YUCCA

The healing properties of the yucca plant, which flourishes in Southwestern deserts and in Mexico have been known for centuries by Indians who used the yucca for medicinal purposes. Next to water, it was the most important single item for their survival.

All parts of the plant were used for food—the flowers, seeds, seed pods, fruit, leaves, stalks, and roots. The concentrated juice of the yucca served as an herbal remedy for many ills. The juice was extracted by steaming or boiling the plant, then taken internally or applied externally. *It was a traditional remedy for arthritis and rheumatism.*

Those parts of the plant used for food were eaten raw, baked, or boiled. The roots of the yucca were pounded in water to form sudsing detergent which the Indians used for bathing and washing clothing or hides, and the early settlers soon adopted this new source for soap. During droughts early in this century, goats and cattle survived on yucca, avoiding the needle-sharp leaves by eating the plant from the stalk outward.

So important in everyday life, the yucca was also used in many religious and social rituals. The wide usefulness of the plant, and its ability to grow and flourish in the extremes of a desert environment, give the yucca a special role in Indian culture and folklore.

B. YUCCA AND ARTHRITIS

Recent chemical research has shown that *the therapeutic agent from yucca is a food supplement containing a high concentration of a vegetable steroid and a saponin.* Saponin appears to be harmless to humans and, through its actions in the intestinal tract, is in fact therapeutic. It has not yet been proven how this yucca extract benefits arthritis sufferers, or how it affects hypertension and other ills, except that *it does improve circulation and reduces abnormal fat content of blood.*

Among the first researchers to become interested in yucca and its ability to survive punishing extremes of heat, cold, and lack of water for long periods was John W. Yale, Jr., Ph.D. A botanist and biochemist, Dr. Yale observed that the yucca contains a high concentration of steroid saponin compounds which were found to act as a combination wetting and anti-stress agent. As older leaves died and disintegrated into dust, the wind would carry these saponins off to other plants and soils, thus helping various desert plants to utilize the scarce water supply more effectively. After he developed a process to extract the steroid saponins, he discovered that they increase water penetration and absorption of nutrients in plants and *accelerate the breakdown of organic wastes by microscopic plants.*[63]

These findings led him to the prevailing theory that *toxic substances or harmful bacteria in the colon, when absorbed into the system, create allergic responses— anything from migraine to arthritis.* Consquently, *an anti-stress agent* such as yucca saponin introduced into the colon might have the same beneficial effect on wastes in the body and be effective in treating arthritis *by improving and protecting the intestinal flora rather* than any direct action upon arthritis.

Strong evidence supports the theory that some forms of arthritis may be caused or worsened by toxic substances occurring in the intestines and absorbed by the body. Yucca seems to inhibit these harmful intestinal bacteria and at the same time help the natural and normal forms of bacteria found in the tract. Most patients who report a reduction of joint swelling and stiffness also suffer gastrointestinal disturbances associated with arthrits. These are gradually corrected by yucca treatment.

C. RESEARCH STUDIES

1973-74 STUDY

The *Desert Arthritis Medical Clinic* began a revival of interest in yucca through a 12-month controlled study at Desert Hot Springs, California. Yucca saponin extract, which is a glycoside combining its steroids with simple sugar (glucose, galactose) was dispensed in tablet form, along with identical placebo tablets, to 165 patients. Half received placebos and half received actual extract tablets. They were dispensed in random order and neither patient nor doctor knew which tablet the patient received. Patients were given six tablets daily over a period of five-six months.

Patients ranged in age from 11 to 92; the majority

were adults, and many were past middle age. The disease had been present for an average of 15 years, and even the youngest patient suffered bone, joint, and cartilage destruction. Osteoarthritis was present in 97 patients, and 68 had rheumatoid arthritis.

Most patients were taking some form of medication—cortisone, gold therapy, or some unknown Mexican drug—and no attempt was made to alter their drug intakes during the study.

FINDINGS. Less than a fourth of the placebo group reported some overall benefit, while nearly half of the yucca group made the same claim. *More than 60% reported overall relief of typical arthritis symptoms such as swelling, pain, and stiffness.* Additional improvements in circulation, skin and hair, and relief from chronic headaches were also seen.

More than half the patients reported some immediate improvement soon after starting the yucca. But there were no sudden or dramatic changes, probably due to the many variables found in such a broad group of patients. Yucca typically works over a longer period of time. It is not absorbed by the intestinal tract but acts indirectly on the intestinal flora—gradually eliminating or reducing harmful bacteria and encouraging the growth of favorable bacteria. From 10 to 20% reported relief from intestinal gas, diarrhea, or constipation.

No allergic manifestations or blood dyscrasia developed, and less than 10% reported some minor one-time or transient complaint, side effects which were difficult to relate directly to yucca. This non-toxic property of the extract is supported historically by the Southwestern desert Indians who have used the yucca as a major food source for centuries.

Based on this early research, other physicians were prompted to try yucca extract, with impressive results. Dr. Paul Isaacson in Arizona reports that 90% of his patients on yucca received some relief from discomfort and sometimes reduced swelling, results he did not see before yucca therapy. Dr. Robert Elliott in California claims that 50% of his patients on yucca gained some symptomatic relief. He noted, that yucca therapy also seems to play a role in reducing cholesterol and triglyceride levels in the blood.

1978-79 STUDY

Further investigation seemed to be called for, so 212 arthritis patients with high blood pressure and high cholesterol levels were selected for an 18-month controlled study with yucca extract. Osteoarthritis was present in 124 patients, and 88 had rheumatoid arthritis.

Again, identical yucca and placebo tablets were randomly distributed in a double-blind study. Each patient received a complete orthopedic examination, and blood tests; all were placed on high-protein diets stressing natural foods and vitamin suplements; all participated in exercise and physical therapy programs.

Placebo tablets were given to 36 patients; 138 received yucca; and 38 were given the placebo for the first one or two months, then yucca tablets for another one to six months, or more. The average patient received yucca for six to twelve months.

Results. As in the original study, over 60% of the

patients received some benefit from taking yucca extract with no reactions, complications, or ill effects.

A significant reduction in blood triglycerides was seen in only 5% of patients on the placebo (17 mg/100 ml average), while 33% of those on yucca showed an average drop of 24 mg/100 ml. A reduction in blood cholesterol was seen in 58% of the placebo patients (40 mg/100 ml average) and 66% of those on yucca (110 mg/100 ml average). Blood pressure was significantly lowered in 28% of patients on placebos (13 mm Hg average) and 34% of patients on yucca (24 mm Hg average).

As these results show, the yucca extract was more successful in lowering these three factors, high blood pressure, high triglyceride and cholesterol levels, than the placebo; and diet and exercise is an effective adjunct to therapy, as can be seen in the placebo group. But more significantly, all patients who continued on yucca extract for six months or more obtained some *permanent* reduction of abnormally high blood pressure or excessive blood triglyceride and cholesterol levels.

The exact method by which the extract works is not yet known. It appears that *yucca saponin tends to break down the high molecular fats in foods* whose absorption contributes to high blood pressure, hardening of the arteries, hypertriglyceridemia, and hypercholesterolemia. Since these conditions are often found in arthritis patients, yucca extract is recommended as a safe and effective food supplment in the treatment of arthritis.

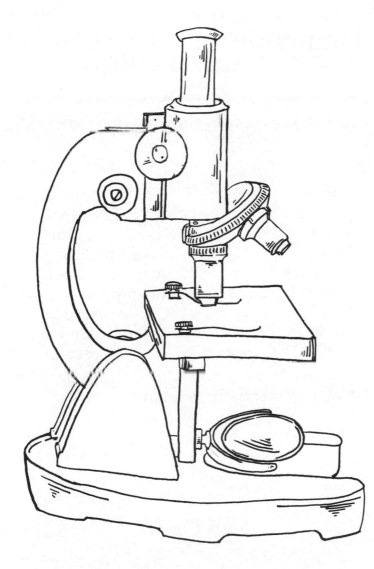

DIFFERENTIAL DIAGNOSIS DEPENDS
ON LABORATORY EXAMINATIONS

Table 13

COMPARISON OF SOURCES FOR ARTHRITIS TREATMENT

NATURAL SUBSTANCES   SYNTHETIC PRODUCTS

Yucca	Aspirin
(Esterene)*	N.S.A.I.D.S.
Vaccines	Gold
Foods	Anti-malarials
Vitamins	Anti-protozoals
Minerals	Immuno-suppressives
DMSO	Cortico-steroids
Herbs	Penicillamine
Folk Medicines	Procaine

* Not commercially available.

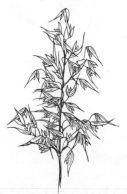

GRAINS FURNISH FOOD AND FIBER

CHAPTER 13

DRUG THERAPY

A. NATURAL TREATMENTS

Has the practice of medicine in the United States become too scientific and less than effective because of the increasing reliance on synthetic rather than natural remedies? *Current statistics show that the medical profession relies 90% on drugs and 10% on other adjuncts for the treatment of arthritis.* Two disturbing changes in medical practice today and the relationship of patients to their physicians point out the problem.

EMPHASIS ON DRUG TREATMENTS

The average doctor today is more likely to be a specialist than a general practitioner or family physician. He relies more and more on synthetic drugs in the treatment of disease. The new antibiotics and other medications which control heart disease and high blood pressure are progressive and medically effective, but the use of some new chemical substances in the treatment of arthritis poses serious questions.

All of these new drugs have shown certain side effects and complications, and *some are more serious than the disease.* The "therapeutic value" of a drug (based on the clinical needs of the patient) must be compared with its "risk value" (the dangers involved in its use) when choosing a drug treatment.

Even though the new synthetic drugs may be more convenient to administer and may cause less gastric irritation, their effectiveness is often questionable when compared with older remedies such as aspirin. They have increased the treatment costs to the individual patient and added hundreds of millions of dollars a year to the total cost of medical care in this country. At the same time *their use has resulted in the neglect, both by the physician and the patient, of fundamental measures in the treatment of arthritis—such as diet, vitamins, exercise, physical therapy, vaccines, and the elimination of foci of infection.*

The typical busy specialist will prescribe a drug which may relieve the patient's symptoms, give him some printed literature and words of advice, and the patient will probably be more comfortable and gradually improve. If he doesn't improve, the average doctor will prescribe a *different* medicine, do some more tests, in the search for something that will help him.

The routine of changing patients from drug to drug is characteristic of most arthritis treatment in the United States—whether practiced by family physicians, specialists in internal medicine, or rheumatologists. There is little difference in treatment whether the doctor is a general practitioner or a specialist except that the specialist probably sees the most severe cases and those that do not respond to the usual drug treatments.

One of the physician's greatest resources is the world's supply of natural substances which can be used as drugs. Drugs from natural sources often are better tolerated by the body and have fewer reactions or complications than synthetic products. Thousands of natural substances are potentially useful in medicine but have not undergone thorough scientific testing or investigation. Chinese medicine traditionally and historically uses over 3,000 herbs and plant, animal, or mineral extracts in the treatment of human ailments; the American Indians use many plants and their extracts for relief of pain and disease. All of these deserve further investigation.

B. PUBLIC DEMAND FOR HOLISTIC TREATMENT

The public is demanding better health care and more natural methods in the treatment of disease. This is being met by the rise in "holistic" medicine nutrition specialists, naturopaths, chiropractors, health and figure salons, weight reduction clinics, exercise gyms, health food stores, and self-treatment fads resulting from the flood of books, articles, and journals directed to the public on health and disease. As this is more outside the medical profession than inside, *there has been a loss of confidence in the medical profession regarding health, disease prevention, and treatment.*

THE DRUG COMPANIES VS NATURAL REMEDIES

A retired physician and medical missionary, who spent decades in Equador learning the art of the Andean medicine men, returned to the United States with 6 natural drugs he had found effective in arthritis, cancer, ulcers, heart disease, infection, and athlete's foot. But no drug company would submit them to chemical analysis, purificaiton, or clinical testing. The reasons were obvious.

In order to guarantee high profits for their stockholders, American drug manufacturers are interested only in drugs they can monopolize—either through controlling the supply or patents or the synthetic manufacturing process. They will not investigate substances that can be acquired, manufactured, and distributed by anyone, with the resulting open market competition and lowered prices to the public. Medical schools, large clinics, and the government (to some extent) are also actively engaged in the research of synthetic drugs supported by the chemical industry, to find new products that can be profitably marketed.

The only solution which seems appropriate is for *the federal government and nonprofit foundations to support and encourage clinical research of natural substances for medical use*. But this cannot be done under present laws covering new drugs. The criteria for analyzing the manufacture of synthetic drugs cannot be applied directly to natural substances, many of which have organic chemical structures so complex that they cannot be adequately analyzed in the laboratory. Animals cannot be used reliably for testing, except perhaps for toxicity, because these anti-rheumatic substances appear effective only on human diseases.

No two patients are alike; no two physicians are alike; and no disease manifests exactly the same way in every patient. The patient seeking medical treatment is a complicated individual with a specific set of problems that must be studied, resolved, and answered.

Human testing, such as double-blind placebo studies, are often misleading as many drugs either have no effect or react differently on the healthy person than they do on the sick.

The only alternative in natural product investigation is careful observation based on the relationship of one patient, one physician, and one natural substance used in treatment. From this point further testing and analysis can proceed. To achieve this, three actions are necessary:

1. *The medical profession must be more open-minded* regarding natural substances and willing to use

them empirically in the treatment of disease, even before all scientific evidence and proof of the mode of action is known. For example: Vitamin C for treating respiratory infection, healing wounds, and preventing common colds; vitamin E for treating arteriosclerosis, heart disease, cerebral and extremity vascular ischemia.

2. *FDA laws must be liberalized to* permit extensive clinical use and testing of natural substances. Their effectiveness and any possible risks can be determined only by collecting the information from thousands of case records of their use in the treatment of clinical disease.

3. *The federal government, private foundations, and educational institutions must make money available for this research.* Funds cannot and will not come from the chemical and pharmaceutical industries who depend on product monopolies and patents on synthetic substances for their economic survival.

C. HERBAL MEDICINE

All races, nations, and tribes use some plants or herbs as medicines in their native cultures. This vast realm of cultural knowledge has not been thoroughly explored and these vegetable extracts may contain useful therapeutic actions for the treatment of arthritis even superior to that which we now employ.

A number of fundamental discoveries already have come from nature: quinine from the chinchona bark for malaria; digitalis from the foxglove for heart disease; aspirin and its natural counterpart from wild wintergreen for arthritis; hormones such as insulin, thyroid and adrenal substances from animal sources. Ephedrine for asthma and atropine for eye examinations are both derived from wild plants.

The drug snakeroot *(Rauwolfia serpentina),* from which modern tranquilizers spring, was first described in the Vedas, the religious writings of the Hindus, and considered a remedy for high blood pressure, insomnia, and "insanity."

Egyptian physicians in 3000 B.C. treated wounds with bread mold; and in 1928, Scottish physician Sr. Alexander Fleming accidentally introduced mold into a bacterial culture, preventing the growth of bacteria around it and leading to the synthesis of penicillin.

D. FOLK REMEDIES

Dr. D.C. Jarvis, a country doctor in New England, used natural methods of treatment in his practice and demonstrated that folk medicine could be combined with modern medical knowledge to treat and cure many of his patients. In one of his books he advocates the use of apple cider vinegar and honey, either separately or in combination, to improve digestion and calcium metabolism—with a total of "eleven beneficial effects on the human body." He received testimonial letters from hundreds of patients who followed his recommendations with relief of arthritic symptoms, indicating that there may be some therapeutic value in his teachings. But we don't know why they help some patients and not others, or whether there is any biochemical basis for their therapeutic actions. According to Jarvis, soaking the hands in a hot solution of water and vinegar for 10 minutes twice a day will decrease swelling, increase joint action, and return grip strength to the hands. His theory is that calcium deposits in arthritic joints will enter into solution when soaked in hot water and vinegar since calcium will go into solution when boiled in acidic water. (Soaking in hot water *alone* will improve local joint circulation, relieve the pain and swelling to some extent.)

Other authors extoll the virtues of natural remedies. Wade (1970) mentions poultices for arthritis, herbs for rheumatism, and root extracts for relieving pain. He is convinced that the high mineral content of many of these herbs and plants would be beneficial to arthritis patients. Airola (1968) states a good case for the natural treatment of arthritis with methods he uses in Sweden: climate, rest, hot therapeutic baths, massage, exercise, diet, withdrawal of drugs, and proper nutrition.

On the other hand William Kittay, former science and medical editor of the Arthritis and Rheumatism Foundation, recommends that patients avoid quack cures, patent medicines, and "arthritis diets." He advises that "it is important to eat right and check your diet with your doctor." *Consumer Reports* published a book on fads and quacks, especially in the nutrition field, and how the public spends millions each year on mail-order nostrums, mechanical gadgets, proprietary and advertised "treat yourself" medications, and certain vitamins and "health" foods in the search for relief from arthritis.

It's foolish to suppose that we'd all be healthier if we scorned synthetic drugs and used only herbal remedies. But many plants and herbs have physiological properties still unknown and may offer great possibilities in developing new and natural medicines and drugs.

BEE VENOM

Stories of *bee venom injections effecting a cure for arthritis* are part of the medical folklore of Europe and Asia. However, early reports of success failed to take into account that arthritis is not a single clinical entity but a multifaceted one. There are, in fact, no reliable clinical indications for bee venom therapy.

In a study at the New York University School of Medicine on the effects of bee venom on rheumatic disease in rats, those receiving bee venom from the first day following infection with polyarthritis did not develop the disease. But *injections failed to alter the course of the disease in those with established polyarthritis* or those treated with the individual components of bee venom. Bee venom probably has a stimulatory effect on the adrenals as it seems to produce sustained elevation of corticosterone in rats and dogs.

Since a national network reported that bee venom may be effective in the treatment of rheumatic disease, many patients are asking for this type of therapy, and many are regularly receiving injections of bee venom from nonphysicians. But repeated injections of bee venom in humans with hyper sensitivity can be dangerous, even potentially lethal, leading to allergic reactions, anaphylactic shock, and even death.

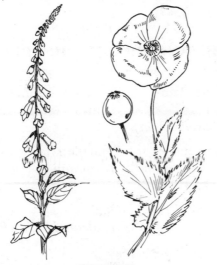

HERBS

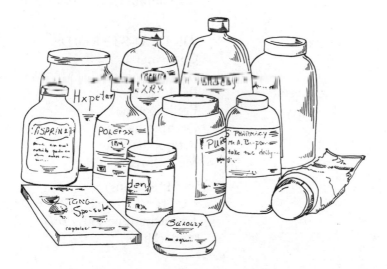

**HERBS MAY HELP AND
SHOULD BE RESPECTED**

Table 14

THE ANTI-RHEUMATIC DRUGS

For Arthritis Pain	To Reduce Inflammation
Aspirin *(Acetosalicyclic Acid)*	Aspirin
Acetominophen *(Tylenol, Anacin and)* *other brands)*	Penicillamine *(Cupramine, Depen)*
Propoxyphene *(Darvon)*	Gold Salts *(Solganal, Myochrysine)*
	Phenylbutazone *(Butazolidin)*
	Oxyphenbutazone *(Tandearil)*
	CORTICO-STEROIDS: Cortisone Hydrocortisone Prednisone Prednisolone Decamethasone Betamethasone Methylprednisolone
	(For Injections) ACTH Triamcinalone *(Medrol)* (and others)

NON-STEROIDAL ANTI-INFLAMMATORY AGENTS
(NSAIA or NSAIDS)

These relieve both **Pain and Inflammation**

Piroxicam *(Feldene)*
Ibuprofen *(Motrin)*
Fenprofen *(Nalfon)*
Naproxen *(Naprosyn)*
Tolectin *(Tolectin)*
Sulindac *(Clinoril)*
Indomethacin *(Indocin)*

To Remove the CAUSES of Arthritis

Anti-biotics   against Bacteria

Anti-malarials   "   Protozoa
  Hydroxychloroquine
    (Plaquenil)
  Chloroquine

Anti-protozoals   "   Protozoa
  Bile Salts
  Copper compounds
  Diiodohydroxyquine
    (Diodoquin)
  The IMIDAZOLE Series of Drugs:
    Metronidazole *(Flagyl)*
    Tinidazole *(Fasigyn)*
    Clotrimazole *(Lotrimin)*
    Furazolidone *(Furoxone)*
    and others

Ascorbic Acid *(Vitamin C)*   "   Viruses

To Reduce Swelling and Stiffness

DMSO
Procaine
Esterene

To Prevent Infections and to Increase Immunity

Arthritis Vaccines

To Affect Metabolism in Gout

Aspirin
Allopurinol *(Zyloprim)*
Probenecid *(Benemid)*
Colchicine

Drugs NEVER Recommended

Codeine and other narcotics
Barbiturates and other hypnotics
Immune Suppression Agents:
   Cytoxan
   Leukeran
   Imuran
   Methotrexate
"Tranquilizers"
Experimental Drugs (Unless there is firm evidence of
   their safety.)

CHAPTER 14

THE ANTI-RHEUMATIC DRUGS

The control of rheumatoid disease obviously requires a considerable degree of judgment. The art and science of treatment are equally important, and clinical judgment is the deciding factor. Until we know all the causes of the disease (and therefore how to cure), we can only try to control the symptoms.

"Nowadays a certain amount of courage is required to recommend a new medicine. They are thrown onto the market almost every day, and one needs a marvelous memory if one wants to remember all of the new names. Many pop up, are praised and recommended by a few authors, and especially manufacturers, and after a short time one hears no more of them. I therefore approached its use with not inconsiderable skepticism—the new medication named aspirin.*"*
—from a speech given by K. Witthauer to a medical association in the late 1800's

Every patient who comes to a doctor for treatment of arthritis hopes to be given a "miracle drug"—something he could take by mouth daily to relieve the pain, swelling, and stiffness of his disease without harmful side effects. The doctor would like to prescribe a medicine to relieve the patients's symptoms, increase his function and physical capacity, and arrest the progress of his arthritis.

But there are three reasons why this optimistic scene does not occur in reality.

1. *"Arthritis" is not a single disease* but a comprises a large family of inflammatory and noninflammatory conditions of the joints (over 100 are known).

2. *Every patient has different manifestations of*

arthritis depending on general health, nutrition, resistance to disease, age, allergy, and the presence of other acute or chronic illnesses. *The treatment of each patient must be individualized by the doctor.*

3. *Each drug used in the treatment of arthritis had its own indications,* therapeutic strength and response, contra-indications, and complications. When selected by a doctor, each must be suitable for the patient's symptoms and take into consideration probable physiological response to treatment.

It should be clearly understood that no drug has yet been discovered which is "good for arthritis" and at the same time "good for the patient." All drugs have some unfavorable effects on human beings. No matter what medication is chosen its use should be limited and then discontinued as soon as possible.

Doctors circumvent this problem by changing to another medication as soon as unfavorable side effects or lack of therapeutic improvement are noted.

A. ASPIRIN

Try aspirin first—but make sure the patient is not already taking it. The question here is whether an effective blood salicylate level can be achieved, as it is sometimes difficult to raise the serum level in active rheumatoid disease. This may be because of low plasma albumin and poor binding of salicylates (50-80% of aspirin is bound to plasma proteins). If the level can be raised above 15 mg/100ml, aspirin may be useful if it is well tolerated.

Aspirin was not developed until the 20th century. A pure chemical drug (acetylsalicylic acid), it was first made by a French chemist working for Bayer, who "rediscovered" its medical value by giving some of it to his father who suffered from rheumatoid arthritis. It was effective in relieving his father's pain, and clinical tests were begun in 1898, with the first medical report appearing in 1899.

Aspirin belongs to the chemical family of salicylates, which are direct descendants of a natural remedy, extracts of willow bark. Over 2000 years ago Hippocrates knew of the benefits of willow bark in the relief of pain and fever; Greek and Roman physicians used it, and knowledge of these plants seemed to be known worldwide, even to primitive societies. The active principal salicin, the North American Indians obtained from the plant "trailing arbutus".

The first English language medical report on the use of willow bark was published in 1763. Rev. Edward Stone dried the bark, made it into a powder, gave it to his patients every 4 hours to reduce fever.

Aspirin was first manufactured and sold by the Bayer Company and other companies could not use the trade name until the patents expired in 1917. Now "aspirin" is a recognized chemical name and can be manufactured by any company. The Bayer Company has strict quality controls and has protected the drug's reputation by maintaining high standards of purity and freshness. *Old aspirin tends to break down into salicylic acid, the same chemical compound used in corn removers, and can cause an irritating or ulcerating effect on the stomach.* Aspirin, therefore should be taken "new and fresh"—preferably with food, milk, or an acid neutralizing or "buffered" agent.

Aspirin is now available in over three hundred different forms and pharmaceutical compounds. Indeed, most "over the counter" preparations sold for pain, aches, fever, and minor illnesses contain aspirin. *Often it is only the aspirin in the compound which has a therapeutic effect.* The purchaser need only read carefully the fine print on the labels to discover that its beneficial effect is from the aspirin content.

In the treatment of arthritis, aspirin has these advantages:

1. It can be purchased in chemically pure form; the patient knows exactly how much medication he is taking.

2. Dosage can be easily regulated.

3. The effect of the medicine can be prolonged by taking eight-hour time release aspirin products. If taken at bedtime, it carries on through the night and can be taken only three times during the day.

4. Aspirin can be obtained in coated or buffered forms, in liquid and in effervescent powders.

Before buying aspirin consult your neighborhood pharmacist about the particular product to be purchased. Regular aspirin users should not rely on cheap bargain brands which may not be fresh.

MODE OF ACTION

Although aspirin is used all over the world and has been prescribed by doctors for 80 years, all of its actions on the human body are not completely understood. Many patients recognize that it is useful in the relief of pain. But it has several other actions *making aspirin the most useful drug of all in the treatment of arthritis and rheumatism.*

Aspirin increases the blood flow to muscles and joints, helping to remove congestion and swelling and bringing more oxygen and healing nutrition through the blood to the bones, joints, muscles, and tendons. The newer, extensively advertised, chemicals for the relief of pain and inflammation do not increase blood flow to the joints.

Everyone who has taken aspirin has noticed the increased tendency to perspire. Aspirin causes sweating, reduces fever in patients with infection and lowers the abnormal temperatures of hot, inflamed joints.

Aspirin blocks the action of the enzyme hyaluronidase (to conserve corticosteroid effects) and the production of prostaglandins E and F, which cause inflammation and fever in arthritis tissues. For the average-sized person, 30 to 40 grains of aspirin a day is necessary to produce this anti-inflammatory effect.

Aspirin prevents the clumping of blood platelets, the little microscopic fragments in blood which cluster together to cause blood clotting and prevent bleeding in injured tissues. But if they clump together around inflamed joints, they interfere with blood circulation, oxygenation of the tissues, and healing. By "thinning the blood," aspirin seems to prevent congestion and thus reduce joint swelling in arthritis patients.

Unrelated to the treatment of arthritis, small doses of aspirin have been recommended as a preventive therapy in patients with a risk of heart attack or stroke. As little as one aspirin a day for men over 20 years of age and women over 40 may reduce the danger of abnormal blood clots or thrombosis.

TRY ASPIRIN FIRST

Since aspirin has the advantage of being the cheapest drug while also being effective, *physicians should use this as the first drug of choice,* while keeping the following in mind:

1. Use anti-inflammatory doses, a total of 2 to 4 Gm a day (6 to 12 tablets) taken in divided doses 3 to 4 times a day.
2. Prescribe a regular dosage schedule, not "whenever necessary." If side effects such as "ringing in the ears" occurs reduce the dose.
3. Give full doses until the patient is free of active disease, or for at least 6-8 weeks.
4. If the patient does not improve within a month's trial period, switch to a non-steroidal drug.

5. A fourth dose at bedtime may relieve morning stiffness.
6. Regulate the dose by effect. Blood levels have a limited clinical value but serve as a check on compliance of the patient (25 mg/100cc is usually anti-inflammtory; 5 to 10 mg/100 cc is merely analgesic).
7. *Buffered aspirin, time release aspirin, or salicylates may be less irritating.*

Disadvantages of Aspirin

1. Patient may be reluctant or unable to take full anti-inflammatory dose.
2. *Elderly patients especially may be intolerant of aspirin, even a dose less than 2 tablets per day.*
3. Side effects and adverse reactions include tinnitis and loss of hearing.
4. Dyspepsia (stomach discomfort) occurs in a third of all patients but rarely with gastric erosions and hemorrhage.
5. Elevated liver enzymes may be seen, usually with doses over 3 gm per day (10 5-grain tablets).
6. Increased bleeding time, hypoprothrombinemia, and inhibition of platelet aggregation are noted with bleeding under the skin.
7. Allergic reactions occur in some patients.

COMPLICATIONS OF TREATMENT

The bad effects of aspirin are all easily detected and reversible. *The most common complication is gastric irritation with occasional bleeding and anemia. For this reason aspirin should be given with food, after meals with an acid neutralizing substance, or in a time release capsule.*

Ringing in the ears and dizziness, mild skin itching and small hemorrhages under the skin can be minimized by decreasing the dosage of aspirin. *Pregnant women should not take aspirin.* In large quantities, aspirin has been shown to lengthen the period of gestation, prolong labor, and probably increase blood loss of the mother at the time of birth.

THERAPEUTIC DOSAGE

The policy of our clinic is to recommend a trial of aspirin in all patients with rheumatism and arthritis- usually 2 tablets 3 times a day with meals plus 2 tablets with milk at bedtime. This dosage is decreased with the patient's improvement, and in no case do we recommend more than 8 5-grain tablets a day for the average size person weighing 120 to 160 pounds. A smaller person should take less; a larger person may need a little more.

COSTS OF TREATMENT

An advertisement in magazines for pharmacists showed that the monthly price of anti-inflammatory and pain-relieving drugs can be an important item in the budget of patients with arthritis and rheumatism. Bayer aspirin, the original and considered by most physicians the purest and freshest, cost $4.21 per month. Compared with aspirin, the relative costs of an equally effective dose of 6 common arthritis drugs are as follows:

Motrin	$15.00 per month
Nalfon	$16.80 per month
Naprosyn	$17.10 per month
Tolectin	$23.70 per month
Indocin	$26.13 per month
Clinoril	$27.80 per month

The chief indication for taking one of these drugs instead of aspirin is to prevent gastric irritation and possible gastric bleeding in some patients. But in general, they have similar pain-relieving and anti-inflammatory effects. *None are "cures" or have any healing or specific curative effects on rheumatoid arthritis or osteoarthritis.*

CONCLUSIONS

Every patient with rheumatism and arthritis should consider aspirin as the first choice of treatment. It is a unique drug with pain-relieving, anti-inflammatory, and corticosteroid conservation effects. It should be taken with food or milk, after meals, or in an anti-acid or time-release form, and in the least dosage effective in reducing pain and inflammation. *The patient's progress should be monitored by regular visits to a physician and regular laboratory studies*—particularly blood counts, sedimentation rates, and hemoglobin tests.

Aspirin is an effective treatment but not a cure.

B. NON-STEROIDAL, ANTI-INFLAMMATORY DRUGS SYNTHETICS

Indomethacin may be added to an aspirin regime to relieve morning stiffness, but it tends to lose its effect in some patients after several months, perhaps because of acquired tolerance. It then becomes tempting to substitute a small dose of steroid at night to relieve morning stiffness.

In the past decade there have been many new agents for use in arthritis. Among these are the non-sterodial, anti-inflammatory drugs— including "N.S.A.I.D.'s" Ibuprofen, Fenoprofen, Naproxen, Tolectin,

Sulindac—with chemical and clinical profiles similar to aspirin, phenylbutazone, and indomethicin. *They have minor side effects not found with aspirin* and fewer major side effects than phenylbutazone or indomethecin. They appear to be more effective than aspirin in diseases in which inflammation plays a dominant role, such as ankylosing spondylitis and gouty arthritis. They all demonstrate the same effectiveness in rheumatic diseases, and their side effects are similar. They all demonstrate anti-inflammatory, analgesic (relieves pain) and anti-pyretic (reduces fever) activity. The combined properties of analgesia and anti-inflammatory make them superior to simple analgesics in the treatment of rheumatoid arthrtis and osteoarthrits, where pain and inflammation play a significant role.

Studies show that each of the non-steroidals is no more effective than aspirin but they may have fewer side effects. Although more patients experienced improvement and comfort, relief of pain, and decrease in joint activity with the non-steroidals than with large doses of aspirin, *there is no over-all statistical difference in effectiveness between aspirin and the non-steroidals.* The difference between the side-effects of aspirin and those due to any of the new agents, however, is significant since anti-inflammatory doses of aspirin (more than 12 5-grain tablets per day) are often associated with gastritis or hearing symptoms.

Advantages of Non-Steroidals

1. *They are as effective as aspirin for joint pain.* Some patients who have had treatment failures with aspirin do well on the non-steroidals.
2. The number of daily doses taken are fewer,

therefore compliance with dosage recommendations may be better.

3. Many patients who cannot take aspirin because
of gastritis or "ringing in the ears" (tinnitus) can
take a non-steroidal drug.

4. Although the non-steroidals have many features
in common, failure to benefit by one non-steroidal does not mean that the patient may not benefit by changing the brand of non-steroidal.

Disadvantages of Non-Steroidals
The non-steroidal, anti-inflammatory drugs do have
some drawbacks:

1. *They are not effective in all patients.* As a rule
30% may do very well and another 30% will have
only satisfactory relief. Approximately half of
the patients will require alternate therapy.

2. They produce side effects in many patients.

3. They do not appear to have an anti-proliferative
effect (altering the progression of the disease).
The result is to control the inflammation rather
than eliminate it. *The patient with rheumatoid
arthritis may feel better but the joint destruction
may continue.*

4. Most have short duration of action and therefore require multiple doses.

5. All inhibit platelet aggregation and may lead to
bleeding complications.

6. *All are more expensive than aspirin.*

7. None have been approved for use in pregnant
women.

8. None have been approved for use in children
other than Tolectin, which was recently approved for juvenile rheumatoid arthritis.

9. All may show cross-sensitivity with aspirin in
patients sensitive to aspirin (Samter's syn-

drome). Accordingly, the new agent shoud not be prescribed for patients in whom aspirin and other non-steroidal, anti-inflammatory drugs provoke asthma, rhinitis, or urticaria.

Indications for Non-Steroids

The principle disease in which they have been helpful are rheumatoid arthritis, osteoarthrtis, anksylosing spondylitis and gout. *It is important* to *make a definite diagnosis in these diseases so that the patient is neither undertreated nor overtreated.* Rheumatoid arthritis may require very potent agents in addition to the non-steroidals, while the same potent agents would not be indicated in osteoarthritis.

Besides knowing the disease the physician must also know the type of patient he is treating. How well does he understand the disease? Will he and his family be motivated enough to follow directions for management of the disease? How much socio-economic help is available? How are physical therapy, rest, and exercise best provided for him? The patient must understand that the use of any drug in the treatment of arthritis should be considered only as an addition to the more general measures of management. *The use of drugs alone, without attention to rest, exercise, and reasonable life-style, will lead to failure.*

Specific therapy depends on the stage of disease, which drugs were previously used, and the presence of complicating factors such as peptic ulcer, cardio-vascular, renal, hepatic, hematological, and opthalmologic problems.

Non-Steroidal Therapy

When aspirin fails to help or is too toxic, one of the non-steroidals may be used. The dose will depend on the disease being treated and the amount of inflammation being present. Following are helpful guidelines for using these drugs:

1. Because some patients are unable to tolerate the drug, always give it with food. If gastric irritability is still present try adding an antacid.
2. When these agents are taken along with aspirin, serum levels are often lower than when the anti-inflammatory drug is administered alone. There may be a suggestion of a somewhat enhanced effect in some instances. But the combination of both drugs may increase the severity of the gastritis, making it intolerable for the patient.
3. All the non-steroidal, anti-inflammatory drugs are rapid acting, but *maximum accumulative effects may not occur until after 4 to 8 weeks or so.*
4. If no subjective effect is achieved within 1 to 2 weeks, or if the patient appears to be getting worse, another non-steroidal should be tried. *Failure* with *one agent does not prevent successful achievement with another.*

Side Effects of Non-Steroidals

All agents may produce gastrointestinal, central nervous system, hepatic, skin, renal, or hematologic disorders. Ocular complaints are also possible. Phenylbutazone can cause hematologic disturbances; indomethicin, central nervous system and gastrointestinal problems.

In a recent study by Dr. Frank Lanza of Baylor University, he performed gastroscopy on arthritis patients taking these non-steroidals. Motrin (1600 mg per day) resulted in the least erosion, followed by Naprosyn (500 mg per day), Motrin (2400 mg per day), Indocin (both 100 and 150 mg per day). Naprosyn (750 per day), and aspirin (3600 mg per day).

Although aspirin showed the most severe pathology, there was also a significant difference between the lower dose of Motrin and the higher dose of Naprosyn, as well as the low and the high dose of Naprosyn. Enteric-coated aspirin proved to be less irritating than either buffered or regular aspirin, although it may not be as effective. Dr. Lanza felt *the best way to lessen the irritating effect of aspirin is to make sure the drug is always taken with food or mixed with antacid.*[48]

Correcting Adverse Reactions

1. Always take with meals.
2. Use antacids if indicated.
3. Drink lots of fluids.
4. Do not take with alcohol, because of increased gastric irritability.
5. Use the lowest possible effective dose.
6. Be alert to side effects, especially in the elderly.

Recent studies have revealed that Tolectin and Clinoril will sometimes produce false proteinuria (protein in the urine), and the physician should be aware of this before ordering a proteinuria work-up.

Motrin (2400 mg per day) has successfully treated acute gouty arthritis, with improvement in 72 hours. Aspirin combined with Motrin resulted in marked (45-80%) improvement in lung capacity of asthmatic patients; Phenylbutazone produced a 25% decrease in lung capacity; and Indomethicin resulted in a modest improvement of 15-20%.[60]

Conclusions

The non-steroidals are extremely useful, and side effects other than some mild gastritis are rare. The patient must realize that side effects are always possible but this should not deter him from trying new drugs.

C. GOLD

Gold salts are the most fashionable of the "presteroid antirheumatics." Of the two types the oil based products is perferred. When rheumatoid activity runs high, *remission can be achieved by the intramuscular injection of gold (½-1 g).* Patients who respond well to gold may continue one injection (50 mg) a month, to be discontinued if disease activity "breaks through." Then alternative treatment, such as systemic steroids, may be necessary.

The disadvantges of gold are so many that most doctors use it as a treatment of "last resort." About 50 per cent of patients suffer complications. These include bone marrow damage with anemia and exfoliative dermalitis, a terrible skin rash.

D. ANTI-MALARIALS

Because of the slight risk of retinopathy with prolonged use, antimalarials have largely fallen out of favor. But *chloroquine* can be very effective in reducing the frequency and severity of joint pain in episodic rheumatoid arthritis. Cloroquine is also an anti-protozoal drug, and it's effectiveness may be from that mode of action. (See the following.)

E. ANTIPROTOZOALS

Small amoebic organisms are present in every level of our biological environment—in water, soil, plants, animals, and human bodies. Fortunately, they are not as numerous as bacteria and only a few cause human disease. The best known amoeba is a pathogenic form of amoeba histolytica that causes ameobic dysenteriae.

Everyone's blood has amoebae antibodies that provide resistance and immunity to pathogenic amoebae. Of rheumatoid disease patients, 70% have positive rheumatoid factors while 30% do not; yet all have fewer amoebae antibodies than healthy persons. *This lack of resistance to amoebae may be a contributing cause of rheumatoid arthritis.* It may be genetic or hereditary—brought on by illness, stress, poor nutrition, or other causes which reduce the body's natural resistance.

Discovery

The late Dr. Roger Wyburn-Mason of England was the first to confirm the existence of free-living amoebae (both pathogenic and non-pathogenic) in human tissues and to identify protozoa as the probable causative agent in cases of *rheumatoid arthritis* and a few other diseases.[62]

He then isolated and cultured the organisms, and further experimentation revealed various antiamoebic substances effective in killing the organisms when added to the cultured cells. These include bile salts, 4-aminoquinolines, copper sulphate, metallic copper, gold salts, emetine, chloroquine dehydroemetine, pentamidine, and levamisole (which contains an imidazole group). Particularly effective are the 5-nitroimidazole group of drugs—including metronidazole, tinidazole, ornidazole, and nimorazole—which possess a wide spectrum of antiprotozoal as well as antiamoebic activity.

Antiprotozoal Treatment

The treatment of rheumatoid arthritis may require only one course of the antiprotozoal drug, along with a reasonably effective anti-inflammatory drug to reduce Herxheimer reaction symptoms. Cortisone should not be given to rheumatoid arthritis patients as it lowers the body's natural resistance to infection—not only to bacteria but also to protozoa which cause the disease.

A rheumatoid arthritis patient should be rechecked in 5 to 6 months, but ordinarily this treatment does not need to be given again for up to 10 months. Time must be allowed for the disease and reaction to the medicine to subside. Treatments should be administered only under the supervision of a physician who has proper knowledge and experience in this field.

Clotrimazole

Clotrimazole is available in the United States as 1 mg suppositories for insertion into the vagina for treatment of trichomonas infections. They are also available as oral tablets. Six to eight are taken, two days per week, for six weeks. In a series of 9 patients, 7 had remission or "recovery" from the active symptoms of rheumatoid arthritis with the use of this drug.

Since Wyburn-Mason's original discovery and successful treatment of many patients with clotrimazole, many other antiprotozoal drugs have been used and tested with varying degrees of success.

Chloroquine, Pentamidine, #4-Aminoquinoline

These drugs have been used with some success in acute active rheumatoid arthritis. Chloroquine, also an antimalarial, has long been recognized as effective in the treatment of rheumatoid arthritis. The results are as favorable, or better, than with gold therapy, corticosteroids, and immuno-suppressive drugs.

Yodoxin

Yodoxin (diiodohydroxyquin) has proved to be one of the most effective drugs in acute rheumatoid arthritis. Some patients find dramatic relief of symptoms in 2 to 3 weeks of treatment, but most patients have a slower, more complete recovery with fewer relapses when taking this drug at decreasing amounts over a period of 3 to 4 months. Three tablets (650 mg) are taken daily for 10 days; then 3 tablets a day for 3 days each month. Routine arthritis laboratory tests are repeated at regular intervals. If remission occurs after the drug has been stopped for a month or more, a smaller second course is given (3 tablets a day for 3 days).

Metronidazole (Flagyl)

Metronidazole is commonly available in the United States by prescription and has been actively used by Wyburn-Mason as well as the National Arthritis Medical Clinic in Desert Hot Springs.

There are two recommended methods of treatment:

1. A large dose (2 g) is given after the evening meal on two successive days, then repeated one day a month as long as active symptoms continue.
2. A smaller dose (1 g) is given each day (500 mg with each meal and at bedtime) for a week; then for 3 days a month if symptoms recur.

This is probably the safest and most economical drug for the antiprotozoal treatment of rheumatoid arthritis.

Tinidazole

Tinidazole is not yet available in the United States, but Wyburn-Mason in England administered 2 g a week for several weeks. It is said to be stronger and have fewer side effects than any similar drug available in the U.S.A.

Bile Salts

Some patients have improved by simply taking bile salts (dehydrocholic acid), which seem to inhibit or stop the growth of harmful protozoa in the intestine. Bile salts are not harmful, cause little or no gastric disturbances, and often improve the digestion. They are taken by mouth for several months at a time. When taken as directed, 20% to 30% rheumatoid arthritis patients show clinical improvement or remission of the disease.

Three bile salt products exhibit the best results:
1. Dehydrocholin. Dehydrocholic acid (250 mg); 3-6 tablets a day.
2. Cholan-HMB. Dehydrocholic acid (250 mg) combined with a very small amount of phenobarbitol and homatropine methylbromide to reduce gallbladder and intestinal spasms.
3. Cholacol. Bile salts (100 mg) and collinsonia root (200 mg); 1-3 tablets a day.

Copper

Copper sulfate has been given simultaneously with bile salts by Wyburn-Mason; it chemically inhibits the growth of abnormal protozoa. For this reason it is used sometimes as an antiseptic in swimming pools for people sensitive to chlorinated water. Rheumatoid arthritis patients often show improvement when taking 25 mg three times a day for two or more months.

Herxheimer Reaction

After administration of antiamoebic drugs (especially 5-nitromidazoles), evidence of rheumatoid disease activity ususally completely disappears in joints and extra-articular tissues within 3 to 6 months. Complete cure is obtained in early cases.

But more commonly *these drugs may induce temporary exaggeration of the inflammatory changes around* the joints and elsewhere; and inflammatory lesions often will appear in a part of the body not previously affected. This may be accompanied by influenza-like symptoms of sweating, fever, lymphadenopathy, rise in ESR, eosinophilia, and weakness lasting from a few hours to a few days. This reaction is also seen in cases of active rheumatoid disease treated with gold salts and levamisole.

This "Herxheimer reaction" is due to the liberation of irritant and antigenic substances from the dying organisms. Since the antiprotozoal drug kills so many of the amoebae, the body reacts to antigens of the destroyed organisms in almost the same way as it responds to exotoxins (poisons) given out by the live amoebae.

Although the patient probably will have a favorable reaction to the drug treatment, the inflammatory symptoms may be painful and disconcerting. Some can be decreased or eliminated by a small daily dose of corticosteroid at the beginning of the treatment with an antiprotozoal drug. Medrol (4 mg) daily for 10 to 14 days usually is adequate therapy when starting an antiprotozoal drug. It may also be combined with 50 mg copper sulfate and 5,000 mg vitamin C daily.

A high-protein, high-vitamin supplement with a small amount of zinc also helps to prevent such gastrointestinal reactions as loss of appetite and upper abdominal discomfort. The anti-protozoal drugs are stopped for 2 or 3 days, then readmitted to the treatment routine in reduced dosage until the patient is able to tolerate them well.

This syndrome is not observed in healthy persons or in rheumatoid patients given antibiotics. *Its occurrence in rheumatoid disease treated with various antiamoebic drugs proves that a casusative pathogenic amoeba is present in the affected tissues and proves that every tissue in the body may contain unsuspected free-living amoebae.*

All these drugs (except tinidazole) are available in the United States on prescription for the clinical treatment of rheumatoid arthritis. If a physician is convinced that rheumatoid arthritis may be a protozoal disease, he can legally adminster antiprotozoal drugs to his patients. However, they cannot be distributed and advertised for this purpose by the manufacturer until more extensive animal and human clinical testing has been done, which may take many years and millions of dollars. But since a relatively few patients would be candidates for this research, and the expense of such an investigation would reduce the profit margin of manufacturing companies, additional investigation into the nature of antiprotozoal drugs for arthritis is presently a project of the new Rheumatoid Disease Foundation. Appendix III.

F. IMMUNOSUPPRESSIVES

The value of immunosuppressive drugs in the treatment of uncontrolled rheumatoid arthritis is still uncertain. *Penicillamine* may be effective when used judiciously, but *how* it works is a mystery. A proportion of patients on penicillamine have less pain and stiffness, can reduce their steroid intake, and often "feel better generally;" but as with the immunosuppressive drugs, side effects such as nausea, rash, and thrombocytopenia are not uncommon.

G. CORTICO-STEROIDS

Introducing a "small dose steroid" regime in cases of persisting rheumatoid activity poses a number of difficult problems. Even if response is good, the disease may later "break through" this dose and require a forbidden high dose—resulting in increased frequency and severity of complications from prolonged high dose steroid therapy.

Even if a low steroid dose is effectively continued, side effects may eventually occur. The patient may become moon-faced, bruised, or myopathic; or he might take his "mini-steroid" for years with impunity, as the majority of such patients do. But serious rheumatoid complications such as arteritic manifestations make temporary steroid therapy mandatory, and a large dose may be required under these circumstances.

Most drugs sold for arthritis are intended to reduce pain, swelling, and inflammation. Due to the "cover up" action of the cortisone family of anti-arthritis drugs, *the patient feels much better even though the disease may gradually worsen.* Cortisone itself is the most notorious offender. A patient taking some form of cortisone can feel well and function almost normally for a time; yet the disease, particularly if it is the rheumatoid type, will gradually worsen until the joint damage is extensive. No corticosteroid drug can control the pain, swelling, disability, and deformities resulting from both the rheumatoid arthritis and the toxic effects of cortisone completely or for any great length of time.

Description

Adrenocortical steroids, both natural and synthetic, are readily absorbed from the gastrointestinal tract and have anti-inflammatory actions (they reduce swelling, local heat, and tissue congestion). They all have profound and varied metabolic effects which modify and reduce the body's immune response to irritants, infections, foreign bodies, and allergy-causing substances.

The *natural corticosteroids* (cortisone and hydrocortisone) *are used as replacement therapy* in adrenocortical deficiency states but have salt retaining properties. *Synthetic forms of these drugs have been developed to increase their anti*-inflammatory effects and to *decrease salt retention, and therefore fluid retention, in the body.* These include prednisone, prednisolone, trimcinoline, dexamethasone, betamethasone, and methylprednisolone.

Indications

The corticosteroid drugs are used in arthritis to reduce inflammation with the associated local heat, swelling, congestion, and pain. They have no direct effect on the *cause* of the inflammation.

Cortisone is used as adjunctive therapy for short-term administration (to tide the patient over an acute episode or worsening of his condition) in such rheumatic disorders as psoriatic arthritis, rheumatoid arthritis (selected cases may require low-dose maintenance therapy), ankylosing spondylitis, acute and subacute bursitis, acute non-specific tenosynovitis, and acute gouty arthritis. It is also used in collagen diseases during a worsening of the patient's condition or as maintenance therapy in selected cases.

Adverse Reactions
Precautions

The lowest possible dose of corticosteroid should be used to control the condition under treatment. When reduction in dosage is possible, it should be gradual.

Secondary adrenocortical insufficiency may be minimized by gradual reduction of dosage but may persist for months after therapy is discontinued. Therefore, hormone therapy should be reinstituted in any situation of stress occurring during that period. Any patient on coricosteroid therapy who is subjected to unusual stress should receive an increased dosage of rapidly acting corticosteroids before, during, and after the stressful situation.

Steroids should be used with caution in the following disorders: nonspecific ulcerative colitis (if there is a probability of impending perforation); abscess or other pyogenic infection; diverticulitis; fresh intestinal anastomoses; active or latent peptic ulcer; renal insufficiency; hypertension; osteoporosis; myasthenia gravis; ocular herpes simplex (because of possible corneal perforation).

Aspirin should be used cautiously in conjunction with corticosteroids in hypoprothrombinemia, which may be evidenced by hemorrhagic spots on the skin or gastrointestinal bleeding. Patients with hypothyroidism or cirrhosis of the liver will experience an enhanced effect of the corticosteroids. *Growth and development in infants and children on prolonged corticosteroid therapy may be retarded.*

Corticosteroids may produce psychic derangements ranging from euphoria, insomnia, mood swings, and personality changes to severe depression and frank psychotic manifestations. Existing *emotional instability or psychotic tendencies may be aggravated by corticosteroids.*

Warnings

Corticosteroids may affect the eyes in the form of the posterior subcapsular cataracts, glaucoma (with possible damage to the optic nerves), and secondary ocular infection due to fungi or viruses.

Average to large doses of hydrocortisone or cortisone can cause elevated blood pressure, salt and water retention, and increased excretion of potassium. These effects are less likely to occur with the synthetic derivatives except when used in large doses. Dietary salt restrictions and potassium supplementation may be necessary. All corticosteroids increase calcium excretion.

While on corticosteroid therapy, especially high doses, patients should not be vaccinated with live or attenuated vaccines because of possible neurological complications and lack of antibody response.

Since adequate human reproduction studies have not been done with corticosteroids, the possible benefits of the drug should be weighed against potential hazards to mother and child when used by pregnant or nursing women, or those of childbearing potential. Infants born of mothers who have received substantial doses of corticosteroids during pregnancy should be carefully observed for signs of hypoadrenalism.

The Cruel Hoax, The Mexican Lure

Probably nowhere in the world are so many arthritis patients seeking relief and being relieved of their money at the same time than in Mexico. Hundreds of patients a day from the border states cross over into

Tijuana, Mexicali, Nogales, Piedras-Negras, and Juarez to get a cursory examination and to buy unknown, unidentified medicines they hope will cure their arthritis.

This has been going on for more than 30 years. It will probably continue as long as patients will travel anywhere and pay almost anything for an arthritis "cure." But the deadly truth is that the "miracle" pain relievers they purchase in Mexico always include some form of corticosteroid drugs.

During a visit to a Mexican doctor, usually no laboratory tests for arthritis are made and no x-rays are taken. A prescription is issued using code words or symbols instead of drug names; it is then filled by a clerk, not a pharmacist, at the local drugstore which is often owned by the doctor himself. The patient is given unidentified packages or bottles of medicine after paying $50 to $200 or more—medicines which, in the United States, would cost a third as much. Transactions are always in cash. American insurance companies will not reimburse the patient because they will not pay for unknown drugs.

The Mexican doctor may claim that the medicines are not cortisone. But when tested by competent American firms, they always reveal a corticosteriod drug (usually hydrocortisone or one of the cheaper glucocorticoids).

Most patients will experience temporary relief of some of the pain, swelling, and stiffness. Large doses of cortisone-related drugs always have an immediate and often dramatic effect on the symptoms of arthritis. *But adverse reactions and dangerous symptoms usually will develop in a few weeks or months.* If these drugs are then stopped too quickly or completely, the patient may go into cortisone-withdrawal shock with weakness, fainting, low blood pressure, internal bleeding, and occasionally even death.

The symptoms of cortisone use and overdose include swelling and edema of the hands, legs, and feet; a "moon face"; excess facial hair growth on women; osteoporosis; softening of bones in the spine with kyphosis; scoliosis; "parchment skin" and ecchymotic red areas on the skin from broken blood vessels; compression fractures of the spine; and even pathological fractures of the hips, arms or legs.

In the Desert Hot Springs clinic some 100 miles from the Mexican border, several patients a year are seen who are suffering from overdose symptoms after taking Mexican drugs. Such chronic insidious symptoms as bleeding ulcers and heart trouble, along with the continued worsening of their arthritis, have only been masked by the cortisone-type drugs.

Other drugs furnished to arthritis patients in Mexico and which may have serious long-term effects are narcotics, tranquilizers, hypnotics, sex hormones, some types of anti-inflammatory drugs, vitamins, ACTH, and methotrexate (a proven drug in cancer treatment which is dangerous and can be fatal in the treatment of arthritis).

Patients should not be lured by the "grass is greener" temptation of drugs so easily available in Mexico. They usually are not available in the United States because their toxic properties have not been thoroughly tested and proven safe for human use. Patients may become aware of the dangers of such unknown drugs too late to prevent their dangerous complications.

Trust your own doctor, not some unknown practitioner in Mexico. Don't risk your health or your life in the mass production arthritis clinics just south of the border.

H. PENICILLAMINE

Penicillamine (under the brands Cupramine and Depen) has recently been made available for the treatment of rheumatoid arthritis, although rheumatologists have been using the drug for more than 10 years. Only recently, however, has the Federal Drug Administration *officially* approved its use for rheumatoid arthritis.

Penicillamine is an analog (of similar chemical structure) of cysteine, one of the amino acids that make up proteins. Although it is a component of the penicillin molecule and usually is made from native penicillin, it is not the same thing as penicillin. Being allergic to penicillin would not mean a patient cannot take penicillamine.

Indications

Penicillamine is indicated for rheumatoid arthritis that is sustained, progressive, and unresponsive to usual anti-inflammatory treatments. It produces good to excellent clinical results in about 80% of rheumatoid arthritis patients able to tolerate the drug. Although its mode of action is unknown, penicillamine has been shown to be as effective as gold. However, most rheumatologists use gold injections first, reserving penicillamine for patients who have failed to respond to gold or have developed an intolerance to it. Penicillamine and gold have similar side effects; but the development of a toxic reaction to gold does not necessarily mean the patient will develop the same side effect from penicillamine.

Of the medications available today, only a few will help slow down the progression of the disease and put the patient into remission. *Both gold and penicillamine are capable of inducing clinical and laboratory remission in some patients. Other medications may reduce the inflammation but do not stop the progression of the disease.*[32]

Penicillamine Therapy

The starting dose is 250 mg each night. As the drug is very slow acting, it may take 8 to 12 weeks for the full effect of a dose to become clinically evident and make the patient feel better. If there is not clinical and laboratory improvement at the end of 12 weeks, the dose is increased to 500 mg each night. If there is no improvement in 12 weeks, 750 mg is given in two doses. If no improvement is evident after another 12 weeks, the patient is considered non-responsive and the drug is stopped.

The maximum time elapsed is one year and the patient must have patience during this time. Some may need only 250 mg to put them into remission, but others will need higher dosages. Most penicillamine-responsive patients, however, will show clinical or laboratory evidence of improvement after the first 6 months of treatment.

This "go low, go slow" regimen is important to help avoid any side effects. Penicillamine has recently been made available in 125 mg tablets to enable the physician to increase the dose at an even slower rate if he wants to; or he may decrease it if a slight side effect occurs (certain side effects are often dose-related).

When penicillamine therapy is begun, all other medications for symptomatic relief are continued, including cortisone. These agents may be gradually withdrawn only after clinical improvement due to the penicillamine has begun. *Several years may be required before cortisone can be discontinued.*

Side Effects

Many patients are afraid of taking medication like gold or penicillamine because of the possible dangerous side effects. But every drug, including aspirin, has some side effects; stronger medications simply have more severe side effects. Generally, lower dosages will yield fewer side effects while still producing a satisfactory clinical response.

The side effects to penicillamine include skin rash, itching, mouth sores, alteration in taste perception, lowering of the blood count, and proteinuria. Serious blood and kidney disorders can occur in some patients, sometimes very quickly, making it imperative to stop the drug immediately. As a result, penicillamine must be administered with caution. The prescribing doctor must be well versed in how to use the drug and which toxic reactions to watch for. Some side effects are so serious as to require persistent vigilance to avoid dangerous reactions. *Blood and urine tests must be made every 3 to 4 weeks and*, at the first sign of any side effect, the dose must be decreased or discontinued.

I. DMSO

Every arthritis patient has probably heard of DMSO and many have used it. A few obtained this medicine from a physician or clinic, while others found it in health food and drug stores. DMSO is also sold occasionally in roadside stands, hobby stores, paint stores, and by mail.

DMSO is a chemical solvent which reduces the swelling, pain, and inflammation of arthritis, injuries, and burns. A 50% solution can be applied to the skin of the affected part twice a day with no more common complication than a temporary skin rash. Dr. Bruce

Halstead has stated that, "next to water DMSO is the safest fluid known."

Veterinarians, who have been using it for years, dilute DMSO with a small amount of water for use on humans, adding to its fame and reputation. Clinics providing intravenous injections and local application of DMSO have sprung up from Nevada to Mexico. *One day DMSO will probably become a common treatment in every hospital emergency room, athletic field, and home.*

The Development of DMSO

DMSO was discovered in 1866; but it was not until the 1950's that it was found useful commercially—as a solvent for many chemicals and as an antifreeze solution. In 1963 the drug was patented by Crown-Zellerback Corporation.

In the early 1960's Dr. Stanley Jacob, a surgeon at the University of Oregon's Health Scientist Center, began exploring the medicinal applications of DMSO. He found that it gave dramatic and rapid relief for such injuries as sprained ankles, burns, and arthritis. But in 1965, when laboratory rats tested with the chemical developed cataracts in their eyes, the FDA ordered the testing stopped and refused further approval.

It should be noted here that isolated laboratory rats are susceptible to infection and disease, and testing almost any drug on them may cause some unfavorable reactions. But veterinarians treating animals for injuries and arthritis find no such unfavorable effects from the use of DMSO. It is used daily on horses and other animals with very beneficial effects.

The Benefits of DMSO

Although DMSO appears to work as a local

analgesic, there is no scientific proof that it reduces infection or inflammation—of such critical importance in rheumatoid arthritis—or that it changes the underlying course of any connective tissue disease.

The National Arthritis Medical Clinic has been cautiously using DMSO for patients for the past two years. (It can be legally prescribed if the physician believes it is the best available medicine to secure the therapeutic effect desired.) The clinic found it particularly useful for intermittently swollen joints such as sudden swellings of the knee or ankle.

It was found to be effective on the inflammation and pain of bruises, sprains, bursitis, and minor insect bites but less effective on chronically swollen joints. It reduces the amount of free fluid in the tissues but does not reduce the swelling of joints caused by thickening of the synovial lining of the arthritic joint. Rheumatoid arthritis, with intermittent joint swelling, will gain the most benefit. Next is osteoarthritis, with occasional pain, swelling, and stiffness. Bursitis, fibrositis, and myositis can be improved. DMSO is most effective when given within the first hour of an acute injury.

Administration of DMSO

DMSO is di-methyl-sulfoxide, a 100% pure chemical solvent that can pass through the skin into the body. When rubbed over inflammed and swollen areas, it improves circulation and helps absorb fluids and swelling, relieving pain in injuries and the swollen muscles and joints of arthritis.

Most arthritis patients apply DMSO twice a day to the skin over the area of pain and swelling, allowing it to soak in until the skin becomes dry. It may also be rubbed into the joints of the hands or feet, which are usually slightly tender and swollen.

A 90% concentration is most often used for various conditions in animals, while 50% to 100% (The 90% to 100% solution passes more readily through the skin) strength is recommended for human use. Stronger solutions may lead to skin irritation and a mild rash, which usually clears up when the drug is stopped for a few days. While most patients notice a taste like oysters and an odor like garlic, this is mild and usually not objectionable.

A small bottle may last as long as a month and is not expensive. If there is any skin reaction, it should be discontinued for a couple of days and then applied less often. If no improvement occurs within a few days, it should be discontinued. DMSO does not conflict with or react with other medications.

DMSO by injection is not yet recommended because there has been little scientific testing for its use or safety. If given frequently or in large doses intravenously, liver damage is the most likely effect. Patients with a good liver, however, are probably safe taking it in the form of a local application.

FDA Approval of DMSO

Although it is not unlawful to buy and sell DMSO, it *is* against the law for the *seller* to make any therapeutic claims for the substance. With so many patients trying DMSO, it would seem that enough medical evidence would have accumulated for approval by the Food and Drug Administration. But this is not the case.

The FDA has approved only one DMSO preparation for the treatment of interstitial cystitis, a chronic bladder infection. An indication that DMSO is not harmful to the body is the fact that 50 ml can be injected directly into the urinary bladder, a very delicate surface, without injury to the patient.

Criticism by the Arthritis Foundation is based on the FDA's statement that DMSO has not been scientifically tested and that medical evidence is only "documentary" (based on the testimony of patients that they have improved or recovered with its use). Before the age of computers, testimonial evidence was enough to approve nearly every common, well-known medicine from aspirin to penicillin. But now the FDA requires medicines to be "double blind" tested comparing a "placebo" group (treated with harmless preparations having no medical or chemical effect) to an equal number of patients treated with the drug to be tested.

J. PROCAINE — GEROVITAL

Procaine therapy is not a new discovery but rather an additional use of a well-known drug.

Dr. Gustav Spiess was the first to discover that procaine had many other values besides its known local anesthetic qualities. But Dr. Anna Aslan, a Romanian physician, extended procaine treatment to patients with arteritis and limb embolisms, increasing its use as an anti-inflammatory agent to treat those suffering from bone and joint disease. By injecting procaine into arthritic joints, some joints that were previously immobile or frozen became mobile and flexible. Most patients had less pain and were able to move more freely.

Over a period of 20 years Dr. Aslan treated some 20,000 patients, and some of then individually for as long as 10 years. Her experience with procaine treatment over a long period of time revealed a number of new benefits. A most important one involved the aging process.

Dr. Aslan theorized that *old age is not only treatable*

as a degenerative disease but also can be retarded, delayed, or at least partially reversed. Gerontologists concur that definite physiological changes occur as the body grows older, with some of the following symptoms: premature aging, with its complex group of symptoms; reduced energy and vitality; diminished hearing abilities and visual acuity; dulled mental functions and loss of memory; *arthritis and other diseases of the muscles and joints;* allergies, alpecia, psoriasis, and aging of the skin; ulcers and bowel disorders.

According to Dr. Aslan, *the body's natural ability to replace cells lost through disease and age diminishes through the years.* Cell regeneration can effect a return of youthfulness to older people, and procaine supplements the body's ability to regenerate the cells. *When procaine is administered properly and in certain doses, it will not only retard the aging process but also relieve chronic ailments, some diseases of old age, and premature aging.*

Description

The generic name for procaine is paraaminobenzoic dietheylaminoethanol hydrochloride, or Procaine HCL (Dr. Aslan named it Gerovital H-3). It is composed of small colorless crystals soluble in water, and is one of the few drugs that completely alters its chemical composition when injected into the body. There it is rapidly hydrolyzed by the enzyme *procainesterase* with the formation of *p-aminobenzoic acid (PABA)* and *diethylaminoethanol.* This may well be the clue to the possible important role played by procaine in the basic biochemical processes.[4]

Dr. Aslan found that *procaine directly affects the cerebral cortex and its dynamics, and acts on the entire nervous system.* The diencaphalon centers, spinal cord, peripheral nerves, and metabolic processes undergo trophic changes from the procaine treatment. Dr Aslan's research suggests that procaine therapy has a stimulating effect on the endocrine glands, which may be its fundamental physiological effect.

Dr. Aslan states that procaine can benefit victims of arthritis; arteritis (inflammation of the arteries); cerebral arteriosclerosis (hardening of the brain arteries); trophic ulcers (ulcers due to improper nutrition to a particular portion of the body); loss of eyesight, due to aging with blurred vision; high blood pressure; and defective heart conditions. It also acts to improve muscle tone, the central activity of the nervous system, and cardiovascular reaction to stress; to increase oxygen consumption; and to help restore the use of limbs to stroke sufferers.

Treatment

In treating the disease and ailments that accompany the aging process, quick results cannot be expected; and procaine is a slow-acting drug. Little improvement is noticeable during the first months of treatment; but by the third month, the beneficial effects begin to appear.

Administration

Procaine can be administered in one of four ways: intramuscularly, intravenously, intra-arterially, or orally. Some methods have greater absorption than others. Intramuscular injection is the slowest method; an oral tablet is economical but must be taken for at least 3 months. Any competent doctor can administer procaine by following the procedures set forth by Dr.

Aslan. However, it must not be given in combination with other drugs.

A single course of treatment consists of 12 injections—one injection 3 times a week—over a period of 4 weeks. Following a 10-day rest period, a second course of 12 injections is given. Then a third series is given, or oral tablets started. Since procaine is non-toxic and not habit forming, the doctor may administer as many courses as deemed necessary. However, the 10-day recuperative period must be observed after each course of injections.

For retarding the aging process in middle-aged persons, a preventative course of injections is given by a slightly different method. The Aslan procedure of 12 injections is followed by a 2-week rest period; then another series of 12 injections is given. This treatment can be continued indefinitely.

Oral administration of procaine follows the same sequence as the injection treatment: 1-3 tablets a day for 4 weeks, followed by a rest period of 10 days.

Dr. Aslan uses a 2% solution of procaine with a pH factor between 3.5 and 4.0, with buffers added. If the pH factor is reduced, procaine loses some of its anesthetic value but its action on the sympathetic and parasympathetic nervous system is more effective. The lower pH factor may be one reason why there is no allergic reaction in most patients.

Treatment Results

One of the most significant results of procaine treatment is that the cholesterol level of almost every patient is brought down to normal. The cholesterol found in the arteries of aging people may be a prime factor in the degenerative disease of arteriosclerosis. Procaine activity on cholesterol and its reduction from the arterial walls may be due to the hydrotrophic action of chloride of paraaminobenzoic acid.

Most doctors treat this condition with higher dietary intakes of magnesium and by increasing the levels of organic potassium and calcium. But the dietary plan for retarding aging symptoms simply does not produce the same results for everyone. With procaine, gerontologists are seeking improved appearance, mental well-being, and reduced blood pressure. In some instances, oral preparations can be used with similar success.

Proper nutrition and mineral supplements in addition to procaine injections is beneficial. Growing old is more than a decrease in certain functions; it is a result of biochemical imbalance. Correct nutrition, minerals, and enzymes are needed for healthy cells and to help bring about a biochemical balance. Dr. Cecelia Rosenfeld, in a lecture before the Humanist Council of Southern California, claimed excellent results from combining procaine therapy with nutritional guidance and many patients recovered with fewer series of treatments in less time.

Doctors have found that procaine therapy has little or no toxic reaction. Another favorable finding is that a patient's abnormally elevated blood pressure may show a steady decline as the treatments progress, with a normal reading in some patients by the end of the treatment.

The Research Continues

Since Dr. Aslan's rediscovery of procaine for retarding the aging processes, over 100 papers have been published on procaine therapy and at least four major studies have been made on its use in retarding premature aging and related symptoms.

From the Charterhouse Rheumatism Clinic in London, *Dr. M.G. Good reported success in treating muscular rheumatism and arthritis with intramuscular injections of procaine. Dr. H. Warren Crow, chief of the clinic, states that procaine therapy is "the most valuable weapon in the treatment of the individual rheumatic patient."*

Studies with procaine in the United States have reported the following results:

Luigi Bucci, senior psychiatrist at New York's Rockland State Hospital, and Dr. John C. Saunders, principal research scientist and assistant in neurology at Columbia University College of Physicians and Surgeons, both concur that procaine therapy is definitely a useful medication for the treatment of aged and psychotic patients.

Dr. Joseph Smigel, director of New Jersey's Pinehaven Sanitarium, reports excellent results in 70 out of 85 "senile" patients. Many of the younger patients were able to leave the institution, and some are even back at their jobs.

Although procaine therapy can alleviate or even retard diseases of the aged and certain other conditions, it is not a "cure all"; there are some failures as well as many successes. *But procaine therapy may eliminate fear of senility and the unproductive existence of people attaining advanced age.* Everyone has the right to live longer, to enjoy an active, productive life, and to view the years ahead with happiness and without the tensions of aging. This may be the "breakthrough" long sought by medical science in its continuous fight against diseases associated with old age.

K. ESTERENE IN THE TREATMENT OF RHEUMATOID ARTHRITIS

A medicine of natural vegetable origin that has been found to have useful properties in the treatment of arthritis has been named "Esterene" by its discoverer, Dr. Lowell H. Somers.

It is a purified form of cocaine hydrochloride, an approved drug used by doctors as a local anesthetic. Its systemic medicinal effects have been studied very little in the last 100 years because of its well known habit forming tendency.

In a treatment series of over 150 patients it relaxed muscle spasm and contractures, permitted better joint movement, reduced swelling and inflammation and improved the physical functioning of all patients 40% or more. No harmful or toxic side effects were noted with this treatment and no patients showed any mental "highs" or habituation to the special form of the medicine.

Treatment of patients was halted by the California Board of Medical Quality Assurance when the California Research Advisory Council and the Food and Drug Administration of the Federal government failed to agree and approve a series of research protocals.

Further clinical investigation is indicated, as the very rapid relief and benefits from this drug appear to exceed those of conventional medications. A preliminary report is available to physicians only at their written request to this author.[2] [41] [52]

L. ARTHRITIS VACCINES

The modern use of vaccines in the treatment of arthritis is a revival of a treatment more than 50 years old. In 1932 Dr. H. Warren Crowe, head of the Charter House Rheumatism Clinic in South London, found that many cases of acute chronic rheumatism in the poorer areas of that city were caused by various strains of bacteria, principally streptococci. He prepared a polyvalent stock vaccine containing killed streptococci and staphlococci bacteria. It was used to raise the immunity of arthritis patients against organisms which can cause foci of infection and some types of rheumatic diseases. The "Crowe Vaccine" is still a standard treatment in England.[16]

In the United States in 1934 Dr. K. K. Sherwood reported that "fully 50% of 674 unselected patients with arthritis and rheumatism, given subcutaneous doses of mixed-virus-infections vaccine, were sufficiently rehabilitated to return to work remained symptom free."[50]

My first instructor in arthritis was Dr. Bernard I. Comroe at the Hospital of the University of Pennsylvania in Philadelphia. In the 1944 edition of his text "ARTHRITIS" he devoted six pages to the use of vaccine in arthritis therapy with an extensive list of references to its success.[15]

No one has ever said that "vaccines won't work" to prevent and relieve many forms of joint pain and inflammation. They just became "unfashionable" or "unpopular" after the discovery of the non-steroidal anti-inflammatory drugs in the 1960's.

In our clinic in Desert Hot Springs Dr. Bernard I. Bellew, a physician with training in allergy and ear, nose and throat specialties, observed that when patients received their "flu shots" or "cold vaccines" their symptoms and signs of arthritis frequently subsided or disappeared. To the method of Dr. Crowe and the information from Dr. Comroe's book he added the use of the current polyvalent influenza vaccine to create a new type of arthritis vaccine. Since then many thousands of patients have been treated, and over 3,000 physicians have been sent information enabling them to use the treatment for their own patients. And, except for an occasional "red and sore arm" and some transient symptoms "like the flu", no patient has had any severe or prolonged reaction or complication. More than 75% of patients with multiple joint pain have improved or have recovered. All of them have been protected to some extent against influenza, common colds, bronchitis or pneumonia, and "strep and staph" infections.

To start the treatment the patient is given a "test dose" of one tenth of one cubic centimeter of the mixed vaccines in a small injection just under the skin. If a pink or red area from size of a dime to a quarter develops in the next 24 hours it shows that the patient has some sensitivity to the organisms involved and will probably benefit from a course of vaccine treatment, which raises the non-specific immunity.

Over the next two or three weeks, at four or five day intervals, four more therapeutic injections of the vaccine: 0.3 cc., 0.6 cc., 0.9 cc., 1.2 cc. are given. Four weeks later a "booster shot" of 1.2 cc. of the vaccine is recommended. This is repeated again in three months, and then every three to six months if the symptoms of arthritis reoccur.

The immunity thus produced is probably not permanent, although some patients go several years without requesting another treatment and many appear to have been permanently relieved of their symptoms and signs of arthritis. Among those was Randy Zimmer, the husband of the beautiful vocalist on the Lawrence Welk show. His recovery was reported in her autobiography, "Norma", and due to her recommendation several hundred patients from all parts of the country have come to Desert Hot Springs for the benefits of the vaccine therapy.

The vaccines used in this treatment are all standard biological products, accepted and approved by the Food and Drug Administration for the prevention of influenza, upper respiratory infections, skin infection, etc. The formula has been changed from time to time with improvement in available vaccine products from the manufacturers. While we mail the latest combinations and instructions to physicians at their request, we find that most doctors will not try the vaccines without personal experience with them or some guidance from the Arthritis Foundation. Their endorsement has not been forthcoming for lack of a "double blind placebo random selection scientific study." The profit in vaccines is so small, and they cannot be patented, so no commercial sponsor of such studies has ever been available. This is another example of conservatism in medicine that often deprives the public of safe but "unproven" remedies.

Some rheumatologists believe that the inflammatory types of arthritis are due to infections, perhaps by organisms not yet identified. Since vaccines are a "natural" form or treatment, building up the resistance to infection by desensitization works in the same way that immunity develops after viral or bacterial illnesses, by creating "antibodies" in the blood to fight infection. Therefore the use of vaccines to build up a general or non-specific immunity in the patient's body is a natural and logical step until some more specific organism can be identified and a special vaccine prepared.

Some clinics and laboratories have had success in preparing autogenous vaccines from cultures of the patient's own organisms, from the nose and throat, for example. And they have reported success in using these vaccines in patients with inflammatory types of rheumatic disease.[38]

A five year retrospective review of our experiences with the vaccine treatment indicates that over one third of patients claim "permanent relief" of their symptoms, one third have temporary benefit — but they must continue to repeat the course of injections of all types and required more specific and additional therapy for their arthritis disease. There were about 3,000 cases in this series, from 1975 to 1980.[10]

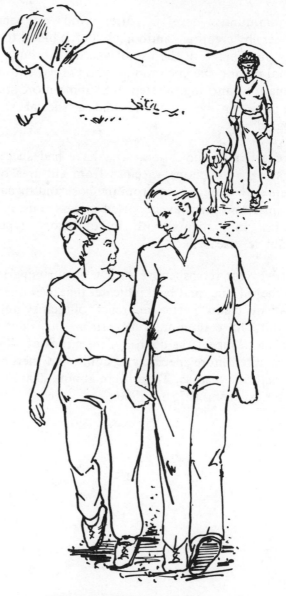

WALKING IS THE
BEST EXERCISE

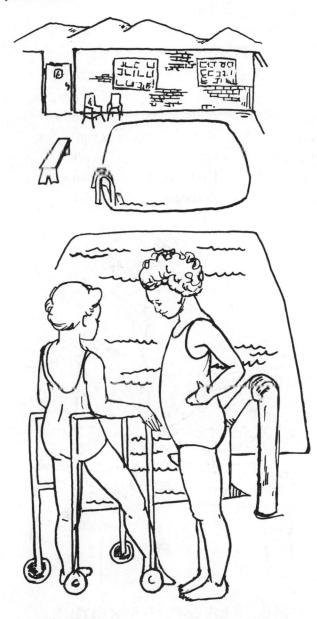

SWIMMING IS A CLOSE SECOND

Table 15

PHYSICAL TREATMENT

Rest	Exercise	Immobilization
Swimming	Activity	Bicycling
Walking	Heat	Cold
Massage	Sex	Work
Play	Homework	Sewing
Dancing	Painting	Music

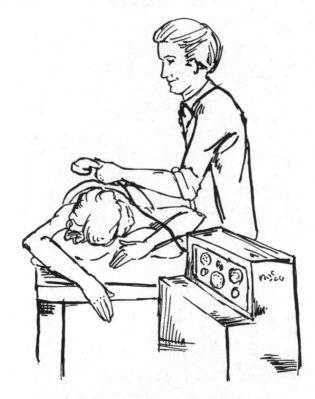

SOME TREATMENTS REQUIRE
REGISTERED THERAPISTS

CHAPTER 15

PHYSICAL TREATMENT

A young doctor, newly graduated from medical school, took over his father's general practice in a small Eastern town. When his father returned after traveling abroad, his son announced: "Dad, do you remember Dan Jones, the banker with a bad case of arthritis?"

"I certainly do," his father said. "His arthritis is one of the most difficult cases I have ever treated."

"Well," the young doctor said proudly, "while you were away I gave him a new treatment. Now he's completely cured of his arthritis."

"Son," his father said sadly, "didn't you realize that his fees for the treatment of arthritis put you through medical school?"

The point is, arthritis is often treated—and perhaps well treated—but very seldom cured. Only nature heals the patient. Physicians and physical therapists must cooperate with the natural restorative functions of the human body, using all medical and physical measures known, to provide the best treatment possible.

Joseph Stokes of the University of Pennsylvania Hospital, Philadelphia, taught a principle that applies equally well to orthopedics and physical therapy. While making rounds with him one day, I commmented on the number of patients who came from great distances—Washington, New York, Canada, South America, and Europe. "How do you always seem to help these patients when all of their previous doctors have failed?" I asked.

He looked at me with a wise smile and said, "I guess it's because I never run out of treatments. There is always something new or different to try for each patient."

That's the way arthritis has to be treated in many cases. You can't promise "cures" but you *can* offer relief. When a case seems stubborn or refractory, the patient will be grateful if you always have something different to try.

A. REST IN RHEUMATOID ARTHRITIS

Rest has always been popular therapy for many chronic diseases, and the importance of rest for rheumatoid arthritis patients has long been debated. But not until World War II was the importance of early ambulation recognized because of the hazards of inactivity.

Investigators recently found that the synovial fluid of a rheumatoid arthritis patient became bloodstained as soon as the patient started walking. After a night's rest, the fluid was clear and the volumes collected were less than daytime collections. Joint temperature increased with even passive and non-weight-bearing exercise. This increased temperature may increase synovial fluid collangenase activity, which may contribute to cartilage destruction and bony erosions. Cooling during rest periods would likely reduce this activity.

In clinical studies of 153 *rheumatoid arthritis patients,* the heavier the physical activity the greater the degree of cystic erosions of the wrist and hand.

In another study, intermittent splinting of the more severely affected arms and hands of seven patients with mild to moderate chronic inflammatory joint disease uniformly resulted in sustained improvement. In fact, patients voluntarily began to rest the less severely affected, non-splinted extremity after improvement in the splinted one.

Rheumatoid arthritis is the only form of arthritis in which rest and immobilization of joints is indicated, and then only in the active, acute, inflammatory stage. When the disease is "under control" and not spreading to other joints, then activity and regular exercise is started and gradually increased.

In a hospital study, 20 rheumatoid arthritis patients were given a minimum of 22 hours of bed rest daily for the first 4 weeks and at least 18 hours daily for the next 6 weeks. A control program involved 22 rheumatoid arthrtis patients given 8 hours of bed rest at night and permitted *ad lib* daytime activity. All patients in the study received physical therapy and therapeutic doses of salicylates, but significant deterioration occurred only in the physically-active group.

For best results in the treatment of rheumatoid arthritis, most physicians subscribe to a judicious balance of rest and activity, including appropriate physical therapy. The ideal program is a "loading dose" of complete bed rest, and improvement is more likely if the patient is hospitalized early in the course of the disease. After 30 days of maximal reduction of articular and systemic inflammation, the patient may gradually increase ambulation and decrease the amount of bed rest.

In general, the longer the period of inactivity the more time required to accomplish reambulation: for example, 4 to 6 weeks are needed for recovery following 6 weeks of bed rest. Patients who obtain sufficient rest to prevent fatigue once they are reambulated show greater improvement and seem to require less medication.

In the early stages of the disease, the patient should have adequate rest while there is a lot of pain and inflammation. This may mean spending as many as 16 hours a day in bed. The contour position of a hospital bed, with the head and knees raised, is ideal for circulation.

Although the arthritis patient can be made uncomfortable by vigorous physical activity, exercises do not injure the joints. Gentle massage, stretching, manipulation, active and passive exercise, walking, and standing may all cause pain but do not make the patient worse; he will be uncomfortable for only two or three days afterward.

B. ACTIVITY

The best news a doctor can hear from an arthritis patient are the word's, "I want you to know that I am *keeping active.*" The circulation of the joints depends on the activity of the adjacent muscles and compression and relaxation of the joint cartilages during weight bearing and physical activity.

Exercise can "hurt", and be painful at times, but it does not cause any injury to the joints.

The best arthritis "cures" are seen in those patients who exercise daily to keep their joints flexible. They do not stop household or personal activities but keep their joints moving. The body gradually repairs and regenerates itself—except for the joint cartilage surface, which cannot be replaced by nature.

Two exercise periods a day are recommended. In the gymnasium, the therapist works with stiff joints to obtain improved range of motion and to increase strength, muscle power, and circulation. The patient usually will notice some improvement in two or three weeks. By the third or fourth week, improvement is maximum (for the time being) and the patient has learned enough about exercises to continue doing them at home.

Swimming is one of the best outdoor exercises for

arthritic patients as it utilizes all body motions while supporting the weight of the body by the water. Walking and bicycling are also accepted methods of exercise if the patient is able to tolerate them. Assisted active exercises and gentle stretching are valuable for improving range of motion in damaged joints.

C. EXERCISE

Arthritis can hurt. And often you'll want to give in to the pain by giving up your normal activities. *Don't.* Your physician might advise a modification of activities that are particularly stressful. But try not to give up anything without checking with your physician first. Prolonged rest periods and days of inactivity will only increase joint stiffness and make it all the harder to move around.

A balanced routine of rest and exercise will help avoid overworking your weight-bearing joints—hips, knees, ankles and feet. Plan to take several short rests during the course of a day.

Have an energy plan. Decide what you need to accomplish during the course of a day. Conserve energy so you can do these things without fatigue or discomfort.

How often do you exercise? To keep joints from getting stiff, exercise frequently for short periods of time throughout the day.

Begin slowly. Try to do each set of exercises twice a day, performing each exercise 3-10 times. If you can, increase *gradually* the amount of exercise you do from one day to the next.

The following exercises were designed specifically for arthritis patients. Not all arthritis patients have the same needs. *So be sure to do only those exercises your physician recommends.*

Aim to improve your posture

Correct posture can prevent pain and stiffness, improve breathing, and keep joints flexible.

Stand with your shoulders, hips, and knees straight, stomach in, and head held high, and walk with your arms swinging freely and your weight shifting from side to side.

Head and knees bent, shoulders curved,
pelvis tilted forward. INCORRECT

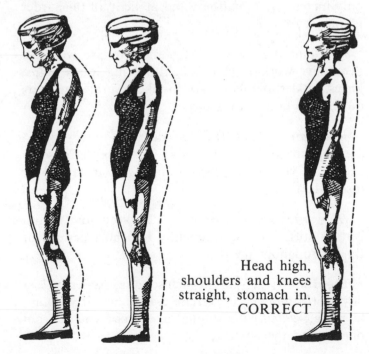

Head high,
shoulders and knees
straight, stomach in.
CORRECT

Sit whenever you can. Standing needlessly will cause you to tire easily.

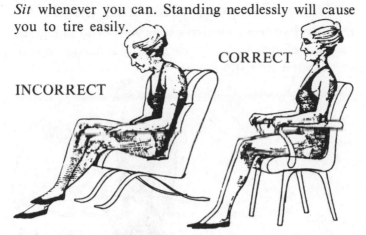

CORRECT

INCORRECT

Sit in a firm chair that is not too low, has a straight back and armrests. When you are sitting, keep your shoulders back, head up, stomach in, and feet flat on the floor.

Lie flat on your back. If you use a pillow, it should be a small one.

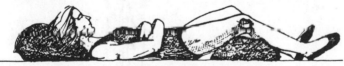

INCORRECT: Knees and hips should be straight. Arms and hands should be straightened out at your side— not folded over your body. Never place a pillow under your knees.

CORRECT: *Sleep* on a firm mattress. A plywood board at least 1/2 inch thick and the same size as the mattress placed between the bedspring and mattress will keep it from sagging.

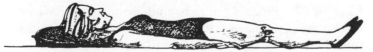

Exercises for your arms and hands

Exercise 1: Raise your arms over your head as high as you can, elbows straight. Then swing arms out, down, and around in a big circle.

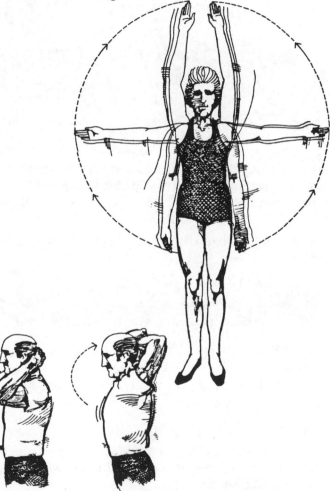

Exercise 2: Place hands behind your head. Move elbows back as far as they will go, and, at the same time, pull your chin in and head back.

Exercise 3: Grasp the handle of a medium-weight hammer near its head. Keep upper arm by your side with elbow bent to a right angle. Turn wrist from left to right, letting weight of hammer swing hand over as far as possible each time.

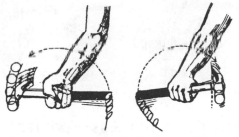

As you improve, move your grip farther down the handle so that the hammer's weight makes you work harder.

Exercise 4: Place hand flat on table. Spread fingers apart keeping them straight. Lift index finger. Then lift all fingers and thumb—while palm remains pressed down.

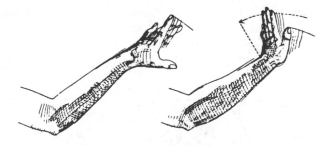

Finally, lift fingers, thumb, and hand, bending wrist up as far as possible—while the forearm remains on the table.

Exercise 5: Open hand, spreading the fingers as you do. Close, making as tight a fist as possible. After repeating this several times, touch tip of each thumb to each finger, pinching firmly each time and forming a letter "O."

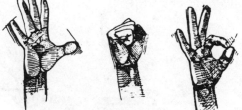

Exercises for your legs and feet

Exercise 6: Lie on your back. Bend knee and hip up toward chest as far as possible. Lower leg slowly, straightening knee as you go.

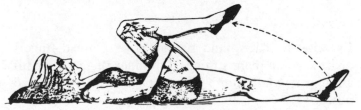

Exercise 7: Lie flat on your back, legs straight and about 6 inches apart. Point toes toward each other. Move right leg out to side, return. Move left leg out to side, return. Keep toes pointed toward each other. Repeat.

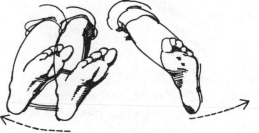

Exercise 8: Sit in a chair with feet flat on the floor Raise toes as high as you can, keeping heels on the floor.

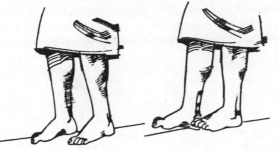

Reverse—keep toes down and lift heels as high as you can.

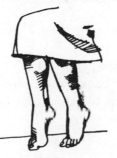

Finally: With feet flat, lift inside of each foot and roll its weight over on the outside, keeping the toes curled down.

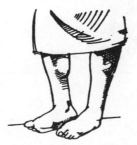

Exercises to improve posture and breathing

Exercise 9: Lie flat on your stomach, arms by your sides. Lift head and bend knees at the same time—as far as possible. If you can, lift your knees a little.

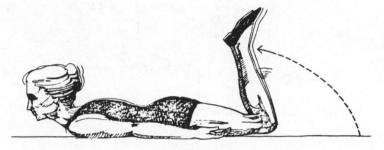

Exercise 10: Lie on your back, knees straight. Lift head, curling your back forward into a sitting position, hands reaching out to your toes. Lie back down and repeat.

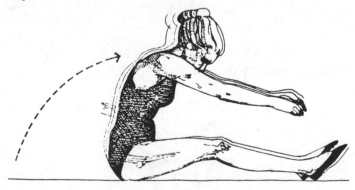

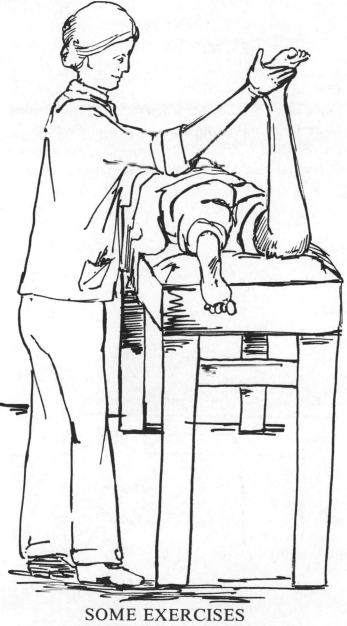

SOME EXERCISES
NEED ASSISTANCE

Table 16

DESERT SPA THERAPY

Climate	Weather	Dry Air
Sunshine	Moderate temperatures	Less Pollen
More Rest	Outdoor activity	Exercise
Special Diets	Physical Therapy	Medical Care

Natural Hot Mineral Water Therapeutic Baths

Southern California

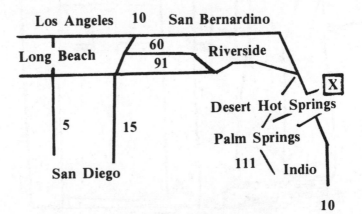

HIGHWAYS

CHAPTER 16

DESERT SPA THERAPY

A. CLIMATE

There is no conflict in medical opinion that arthritis is affected by the climate and by weather changes. Any patient with a swollen and tender joint becomes a "weather prophet" when a storm is approaching, he can "feel it in his bones". This phenomenon is due more to barometric pressure than to humidity or temperature, although cold and damp weather is known to aggravate most types of chronic arthritis, the air is "lighter" when the barometer falls before a coming storm. The swelling of joints increases from less weight of air on the body. This slight difference in air pressure on arthritic articulations creates the typical pain associated with adverse changes in the weather.

The dry and generally warm temperatures of the deserts and semi-arid areas of the Southwest, California, Arizona and New Mexico, have long been meccas for arthritic patients from the colder and more moist regions of the United States. Freedom from industrial dusts, smog and pollens help the sufferers who also have allergic problems.

At our Clinic patients frequently relate in their medical histories, "My doctor says he has done all he can for me. He suggested I try a warm, dry desert climate for awhile." In a few weeks they are usually dramatically improved. Their health is better from both the favorable climate and the changes in life styles and occupations. They are away from the stresses of work and family pressures. They rest better, exercise more, take hot mineral baths, watch their diets, smoke less—or quit at our urging, take vitamins, drink the natural mineral water, and reduce their consumption of caffeine and alcoholic beverages.

Their arthritis is relieved as their health improves. They are FIGHTING BACK AGAINST ARTHRITIS. It is no wonder then, with medical treatment and supervision, the majority of visitors to the desert area who have symptoms and signs of arthritis make "great progress" in just two or three weeks. Some persons, those who are retired or financially able, move permanently to the desert climate to enjoy better health the rest of their lives.

For some unknown reasons, warm climates such as the tropics, damp and rainy areas and low altitudes along the coasts seem to aggravate the symptoms of most arthritis patients.

B. DESERT HOT SPRINGS, CALIFORNIA

The discovery of Desert Hot Springs began with Cabot Yerxa, the first white man to come and live in the area in 1913. He is credited with the finding of the natural hot mineral water—although the Indians have known of these natural spas for generations and found the original "Palm Springs". Cabot Yerxa's Indian Pueblo Museum is now a California Historical Landmark and a tourist attraction for the visitors.

L.W. Coffee established the first public bathouse in 1932. Since then a health resort city of 6,000 people has been built with hotels, motels, apartments, and recreational vehicle parks for those seeking relief from arthritis. The little city has become the residence of many people who have been seeking a healthy climate and a retirement community that is typically American.

My personal associations with the desert area began almost thirty years ago when local citizens helped me start a clinic for afflicted children, now the Angel Crippled Childrens Foundation, a 50 bed residential home for handicapped individuals. Next came a free clinic for the physically handicapped, the Desert Crippled Childrens Clinic. The medical and orthopedic work changed gradually from treating only children, particularly those with arthritis, to accepting patients of all ages. The DESERT ARTHRITIS MEDICAL CENTER, INC., a California non-profit corportation, and the non-profit community DESERT ARTHRITIS MEDICAL CLINIC were formed in 1967.

Along with my training and experiences in orthopedic surgery I maintained an interest and studied the treatment of arthritis patients while practicing in Colorado, Alabama, Mississippi, Pennsylvania, New York, the South Pacific and other parts of California. I have never seen children and adults improve so fast in health and strength and recover so completely from illnesses, injuries and chronic physical handicaps as they do in Desert Hot Springs, particularly with the use of the natural hot mineral waters for therapeutic baths and underwater exercising.

The abundance of natural hot mineral waters in Desert Hot Springs does not depend on rainfall. It is a volcanic byproduct of the cooling of the magma, the hot liquid center of the earth. The hot "pelagic" water comes to the surface via faults or cracks in the earth's crust. Along the northern borders of the city a line of rock slides reveals the San Jacinto branch of the famous San Andreas fault. Wells drilled south of this line produce an inexhaustible supply of natural hot

water, containing minerals beneficial to the human
body and with no unpleasant odor or taste. It is
considered to be a "very valuable natural health
resource." Some authorities have called it the finest
natural hot mineral water in the United States, and the
supply is unlimited.

The location of Desert Hot Springs, just 15 minutes
from Palm Springs and the Palm Springs Airport, the
nearby highway Interstate 10, and about two hours
drive east of the city of Los Angeles, makes the area
one of the most accessible health resort regions in this
country.

C. WEATHER

Contrary to many beliefs, constant warm weather
both day and night is not beneficial to good health.
Neither is constant cold weather. Alternating
temperature of warm days and cool nights are the most
physiological and stimulating to mental and physical
activity of the human body. The desert heat is tolerated
because the air is so dry. Any shade and the slightest
breeze compensates for the heat of the sun. Of course,
with modern electric and gas heating and air
conditioning the coldest days of winter and the hottest
days of summer can be tolerated. Many arthritis
patients prefer the summer, "because the heat makes
me feel so good", some of them say. High winds can be
an inconvenience, as in any desert area, but Desert Hot
Springs is above the valley floor and relatively free of
sand and dust storms.

D. SUNSHINE

One of the least understood and most abused values
of desert living lies in the natural rays of the sun, which

emits three types of radiation useful to mankind: light, heat and ultraviolet radiation.

Light. Light is beneficial to the eyes. The eye muscles are strengthened by accommodation to the brilliant reflection of the sun off the desert floor. Very few outdoor workers wear eyeglasses except perhaps for reading, and many whose eyes are only slightly weak usually notice some improvement in their vision.

Sunglasses offer protection from the wind and midday glare, and Polaroid lenses reduce reflection so dangerous to daytime driving. After a few weeks at the desert, many people discard their sunglasses except when hiking or driving.

Heat. Heat from the sun's rays should be used in moderation. Light-colored, loose clothing permits evaporation from the skin and air circulation. Exercise and recreation should be avoided in the hottest part of the day.

Yet, because of the dry air, winds, and availability of shade, I have never treated a case of heat prostration in the desert in all of the years I have practiced here. Heat stroke in the desert is chiefly from dehydration and physical exertion in the blazing midday sun. People stalled on the road should stay with their vehicles in the shade, avoiding the sun's heat and physical exertion until rescued.

Ultraviolet light. The sun's ultraviolet radiation provides a beneficial, protective, and beautiful tan on human skin. Light tanning increases the skin's strength and resistance, provides protective coloration against the sun's strong rays, stimulates the formation of red and white blood cells, and helps build resistance against infection.

The ability of ultraviolet light to create vitamin D and prevent rickets in children is well known. But less appreciated is the fact that it also improves calcium metabolism in adults, facilitates recovery from arthritis, and helps overcome osteoporosis (particularly common in women past the age of menopause).

The frequent association of healthy, tanned skin and well-calcified bones and joints is too common to be mere coincidence. Conversely, pale white, flabby skin is often associated with osteoporosis and the lack of calcium adjacent to the joints in atrophic arthritis or rheumatoid arthritis.

Children respond to the desert climate more quickly than adults, as indicated by x-rays taken three to six months after they come to the desert for treatment. Those with fractures seem to heal more quickly in the desert because their calcium metabolism is fostered by the ultraviolet rays of the sun.

Sunbathing should be maintained on a regular schedule until a light or moderate tan is obtained. Avoid rapid tanning or sunburn—not only because of the pain and inconvenience but because of the toxic substances released into the body by burned skin.

The best times for sunbathing are 9 to 11 in the morning and 2 to 4 in the afternoon to avoid the direct rays of the midday sun. From 15 to 30 minutes a day is sufficient to obtain a good tan. The face and eyes— which receive sufficient sun during everyday activities—should be shaded. The body should be exposed evenly, for 5 to 10 minutes on the front, back, and each side.

Sunbathing should be done on a regular basis, at least every two or three days, so the beneficial effect of one day's tan will be added to the next before it has a chance to fade. Suntan preparations are not necessary. A sunscreen lotion may be used for persons who have a blond or very sensitive skin, particularly on the face, hands and arms. A quick dip in a swimming pool will cool the skin and prevent excessive dryness.

Excessive tanning should be avoided. Skin cancers on the back of the hands and on the face are more common in those who have spent long years in the sun without protection. Excessive bathing with soap should also be avoided, as it removes the skin's natural oils and prevents the formation of natural vitamin D. Except for areas of perspiration, a soapy bath should not be necessary more than once or twice a week.

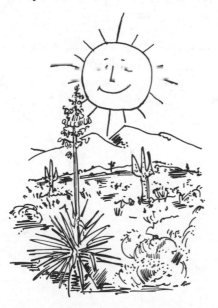

THE DESERT IS ONE OF NATURES CURES

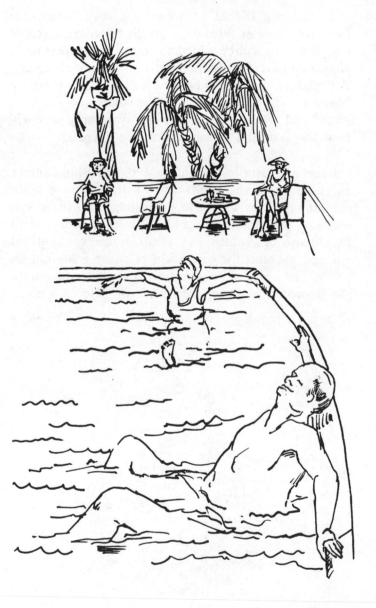

COMBINE REST WITH RECREATION

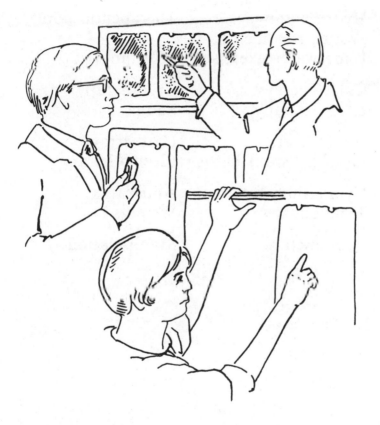

GET MORE THAN ONE
MEDICAL OPINION

Table 17

PHYSICAL THERAPY

Hydrotherapy (Water treatment)	Therapeutic pools
Underwater exercises	Whirlpool
Cold Therapy	Cryotherapy
Heat Therapy	Sauna
Ultrasound	Diathermy
Paraffin (wax) baths	Electrotherapy
Gymnasium treatment	Apparatus
Traction	Weights
Acupuncture	Manipulation

CHAPTER 17

PHYSICAL THERAPY

The human body responds to the natural forces of heat and cold, water, air, electricity and the "laying on of hands", which is massage or manipulation. These constitute natural methods of treatment applied to the outside of the body and are contained in the term "physical therapy", compared with medicines as "internal therapy", or injections and surgery which are "invasive therapy". The term applies specifically to treatments ordered by your doctor, who may be your personal physician, an internist, a rheumatologist, an orthopedic surgeon or a specialist in the field of "physical medicine" with the often confusing name of "physiatrist". He writes the orders or the prescription which contains the diagnosis, the specific "modalities"—another name for treatments—and their duration and frequency. Then he sees the patient from time to time to check on progress and modify the orders as needed. The doctor usually does not give the treatments personally except in the cases of acupuncture or manipulation.

All types of arthritis improve with the use of physical therapy. The degree of success depends upon:

1. The knowledge and experience of the physician.
2. The skill of the physical therapy technician.
3. The cooperation of the patient.
4. The length of time the treatments are given.

DON'T EXPECT MIRACLES

A question always asked of patients is, "How long have you had arthritis" The answer may be, from a few weeks to many years. The length of time to reach a stage of recovery or maximum relief of symptoms from arthritis, even with the best of efforts, may be equally long. After a course of therapy under professional supervision many patients and their families learn enough to carry on similar care at home.

A. HYDROTHERAPY

This is the medical term for "water treatment," probably the oldest form of relief for arthritis and rheumatism. Every natural hot springs area in the world has its history and tradition of the benfits from bathing in hot pools, drinking the water, breathing the vapors and as cleansing agent for douches and enemas. It is also valuable as an exercise medium in therapeutic and swimming pools. The Romans had their public bath palaces, the American Indians used natural hot springs, and every area of volcanic activity seems to have some hot mineral water facility. In this country most have fallen into disuse except from a few well known spas still patronized by tourists and persistent health speakers. Saratoga Springs N.Y., Warm Springs, Georgia and Hot Springs National Park, Arkansas have lost most of the mystique. On my world travels only in Russia did I find hydrotherapy institutions still being used to the fullest possibilities — and free to members of the labor unions and the public under their health system. Rehabilitation in the Soviet Union is a complete program, from healing of the disease or injury until the worker is able to return to employment in his previous job or to one made for him by his industry or field of work.

Dr. J. H. Kellog at the Battle Creek Sanitarium wrote in 1901 in his monumental book, "RATIONAL HYDROTHERAPY", "Modern scientific research has placed upon a sure foundation the great truth, dimly recognized by the earliest physicians and wholly lost sight of during the Dark Ages, that healing power is not possessed by physicians, nor by remedies, but that the curative process is simply a manifestation of the forces which dwell within the body and which are normally occupied in creating and maintaining the organism. In other words, THE BODY MUST HEAL ITSELF.

"Water, applied externally or internally, at such temperatures as may be required is a natural agent more capable than any other of cooperating with the healing powers of the body in resisting the onset and development of pathogenic processes. There is no other remedy by which the movements of the blood and the blood supply, both general and local, and in fact every form or vital activity, may be so readily controlled as by hydriatic applications."

He went on to say, "Water is recognized as without doubt one of the most valuable of all natural agencies. It is best employed in connection with the use of electricity, massage and medical gymnastics.

"Rational diet is as essential in the treatment of the majority of cases of acute and chronic disease as is water. The regulation of exercise, dress and other habits of life is also a matter of paramount importance." He recommended that patients with arthritis and rheumatism should abstain from the use of tea, coffee, tobacco and alcoholic beverages. He strongly advocated the use of natural foods and vegetarian diets.

Are today's physicians, full of the latest knowledge in scientific medicine and charmed by the multitude and strength of synthetic drugs, obtaining less than the best possible recoveries of their patients by neglecting these fundamental truths and methods of hydrotherapy and health?

B. THE ORIGIN OF MINERAL WATERS

Naturally hot mineral waters are not the result of rainfall but are the by-product of the cooling off process of the deep volcanic areas of the earth.

These are "pelagic waters", forcing their way to the surface through fissures in the mantle of rock—the same faults that are active in volcanos and earthquakes. They contain little or no organic matter, are safe and pure to drink, and contain high mineral concentrations according to the type and composition of the rock layers through which they flow. They may be above boiling, producing steam or geyers, or flow gently under deep layers of broken rock and sand, requiring wells to reach the best depths and temperatures.

Desert Hot Springs have the latter type of naturally hot mineral water strata. Very fortunately this pure water of volcanic origin has no sulfur odor or chemical taste. Yet all of the minerals present are useful and necessary in the human body and especially beneficial to arthritis patients. Why is it not bottled and sold? Because it loses some of its mineral content as it cools as a deposit on the pipes, machinery and containers. This is also the reason that the best mineral water pools are the ones fed directly from the wells and pumps at a naturally warm temperature and do not have to be artificially reheated. But even the city drinking water is better than in almost any other city in the world.

C. TREATMENT TECHNIQUES FOR HOT MINERAL WATER BATHS

Patients who are seeking relief in the shortest time possible should go into the hot waters three times a day, mornings, afternoons, and before retiring at night if they are staying in a hotel, motel or recreational vehicle park that has its own naturally hot pools. The water temperatures of the therapeutic pools should be between 102 and 105 degrees Farenheit. In other words, the temperature should be higher than that of the body to stimulate the circulation and raise the warmth of the muscles and joints to the same level as the interior of the body. For every 10 degrees of increase in temperature, of the skin on the hands or feet for example, there is a 50% increase in circulation of the blood and of metabolism in the bones and joints.

THE THREE DIP METHOD

GO IN THE HOT POOL THREE TIMES, THREE TIMES A DAY

1. Soak in the natural hot therapeutic pool 5 to 10 minutes.
2. Get out and allow the air to cool your body.
3. Go in the hot pool a second time, for only 5 minutes.
4. Get out and walk until cool and a little tired, or do underwater exercises and swim, if you can, in the swimming pool.
5. Go in the hot pool a third time, for only 5 minutes.
6. Get out, dry thoroughly, and lie down for a little rest.

D. WHIRLPOOLS AND UNDERWATER EXERCISES

Active exercises in the water and the motion of whirlpool jets of water and air stimulate the circulation and help bring all parts of the body to the same temperature. (This is the reason a deep therapeutic pool is more effective than the usual bathtub in which the water can cover only part of the body at a time.) In addition the movement of the water over the skin stimulates the nerve endings, much like light massage, and the nervous system then releases "endomorphins", the hormones which decrease pain.

E. COLD THERAPY — CRYOTHERAPY

The use of cold is valuable during the acute and inflammatory stages of arthritis. It may be administered by cold moist packs, ice or chemical cold packs over moist towels or by ice cold water. Treatment is for five to ten minutes followed by a slow warming to normal room temperatures. In Europe ice water foot baths, about ten feet long are used. The patient walks through the foot bath very slowly. Then the feet are dried and wrapped in towels to regain their natural temperature. The pain is relieved and the swelling and inflammation are reduced considerably. The treatments are given once a day.

In studies at Germantown Medical Center, Philadelphia, 100 patients with painful knee joints from rheumatoid arthritis were treated with either hot or cold packs for several weeks. They were studied for range of knee motion, reduction in swelling, strength, duration of sleep at night and relief of pain.

> 50 patients improved from 10 to 50%
> and preferred heat.
> 32 patients improved from 30 to 50%
> and preferred cold.
> 18 patients improved from 10 to 40%
> but could tell no difference
> between the benefits of heat or cold

Nalozone, an opiate antagonist, blocked the efficacy of the cold therapy in 20 out of 22 patients. This indicates that cold administration produces its anti-pain response by the release of naturally occurring endomorphins.

Alternating hot and cold packs are also useful in arthritis after the acute inflammatory stage is past. Sister Elizabeth Kenny demonstrated this to me in the treatment of the pain and muscle spasm of poliomyelitis patients when I was the chief of the medical staff at the Sister Kenny Hospital in El Monte, California before coming to Desert Hot Springs. The exchange of heat and cold produces a "pumping" function, on the blood vessels and tissue fluid of the joint and under the skin — bringing increased blood supply and oxygen to the inflamed areas and expelling lactic acid, carbon dioxide and products of cell damage and inflammation.

A QUESTION FREQUENTLY ASKED "ARE HOT BATHS EVER HARMFUL?"

In 25 years or more of treating patients of all ages in Desert Hot Springs I have never known of a case of a patient collapsing in a hot pool or having any sort of an attack or reaction afterwards that was at all serious.

Naturally, if a patient stays in hot water too long he may experience weakness, nausea and palpitation of the heart. But this subsides with a little rest. The heart beat increases its rate in some persons when their body is very warm. And they may feel "like the heart is pounding". This may be compared to an automobile going down hill — the engine goes faster and is more noisy, but it is working less hard than when the car is on the level. Similarly, the heart in a overly warm body goes faster but is under less strain, as the heat has "opened up" more blood vessels and capillaries and the blood flows with less resistance throughout the body. Hot therapeutic baths help reduce high blood pressure, decrease hardening of the arteries, relieve angina pain and stop muscle cramps. Repeated hot baths and underwater exercises are beneficial to patients who have poor circulation to the joints, as in arthritis, and also for patients who have had strokes or heart attacks.

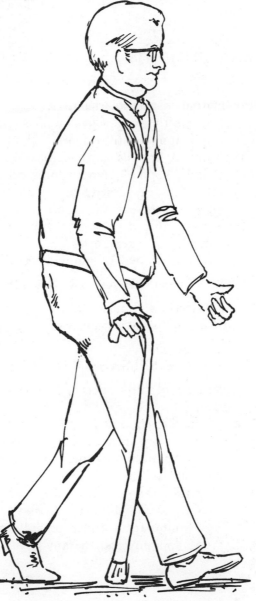

DON'T BE ASHAMED TO USE A CANE

Table 18

SPINAL ARTHRITIS AND MANIPULATION

TYPES OF SPINAL ARTHRITIS

Rheumatoid disease of the spine
    Destroys the joint cartilages, osteoporosis
Ankylosing spondylitis
    Ligament fibrosis and calcification
    ("Bamboo spine", hypertrophic calcification)
Osteoarthritis, degenerative arthritis
    Spurs, exostoses, osteosclerosis
Intervertebral disc disease, infection, herniation,
    calification, degeneration
Combinations of two or more types.

PREVENTION OF SPINAL ARTHRITIS

Avoid: Infections, injuries, chronic disease,
    dietary deficiencies and excessive physical
    strain.

TREATMENT OF SPINAL ARTHRITIS

1. Treatment of the underlying bone and joint
   disease.
2. Manipulative treatment to relieve stiffness,
   correct deformities, reduce subluxations,
   decrease pain,remove nerve root pressures
   and improve function.
       Office manipulations
       Cervial and lumbar traction
       Manipulation under general anesthesia.
3. Exercise and physical therapy.

CHAPTER 18

SPECIAL TECHNIQUES — Spinal Arthritis

A. ULTRASOUND

Ultrasound therapy is used for the most affected and painful joints. Micromassage of ultrasound breaks up adhesions, dissolves excess calcium deposits, and improves circulation.

Dr. Frank Zach, physical medicine specialist at the Kaiser Foundation Hospital in San Francisco, showed that ultrasound could be used safely even on children. In the acute and convalescent stages of disease it helps reduce chronically painful, tender, and swollen joints, muscle contractions, stiffness, and fibrosis. Ultrasound should be given two or three times a week, as one treatment a week doesn't give a prolonged effect.

At the Army-Navy Hospital in Hot Springs, Arkansas, ultrasonic therapy was found to surpass all other methods of physical therapy in the relief of pain and spasm. The proper dose did not aggravate the pain and swelling in acute cases as did some other methods. Beneficial effects were decreased pain and spasm and increased range of motion.

The nerve roots and trunks were treated with ultrasonic therapy as well as the localized joints and muscles. Peripheral joints showed a decrease in inflammation, swelling, and effusion followed by an increase in motion.

The application of ultrasonic waves in degenerative joint disorders should be radicular, treating the following nerve roots:

INVOLVED JOINT . . . . . NERVE ROOT
Hip . . . . L.3 to L.5
Knee . . . . TH.12 to L.3
Ankle . . . . S.1 to S.4
Shoulder . . . . C.4 to TH.2
Elbow . . . . .C.4 to C.6
Wrist and Fingers . . . . C.5 to TH.2

Two thirds of the time expended should apply to the nerve root and one third to the affected joint. The dosage varies, according the the weight of the patient, between 8 and 15 watts. The interval between treatments depends upon the symptoms: acute or subacute cases are treated weekly with a higher dosage. As in all other forms of treatment, the course of the reaction varies from patient to patient and the dosage must be individualized.

Osteoarthritis of the spine is also improved by ultrasonic waves. Cervical spondylitis, usually so difficult to influence, is usually greatly improved (the pain as well as active and passive movements) by extensive ultrasonic therapy in the majority of cases.

B. SPINAL ARTHRTIS AND MANIPULATION

ARTHRITIS OF THE SPINE is one of the most common disabilities of old age.

Yet it can begin at any age. It may be due to injury, disease, dietary deficiency, or any combination of these three causes.

The lower back, the lumbar spine, is usually affected

first. The neck is second in frequency of attack, and if the condition is progressive, then both areas will probably be affected. The chest area may be involved, the thoracic spine, but this condition may be "silent", that is, the patient may become stooped and "round shouldered" but have little or no pain.

a. STIFFNESS OF THE NECK OR LOWER BACK is usually the first symptom of arthritis of the spine. The patient notices difficulty in picking up objects on the floor, or turning the head to right or left while driving. There may be a gradual onset of pain with each effort at bending or lifting. The discomfort may be easily relieved, at first, by moving around to increase the circulation and "loosen up the joints". Heat helps, so does aspirin. And the changes may be so slow that the patient thinks, "This is just old age creeping up the back."

But these complaints and physical signs are really the first indications of changes in the vertebrae that should have the attention of a doctor, a medical and spinal examination, blood studies and x-rays to determine the true diagnosis and to start the appropriate treatment.

b. PREVENTION IS BETTER THAN

TREATMENT

EARLY TREATMENT MAY ARREST SPINAL

ARTHRITIS
or

AFFECT A CURE

c. THE PREVENTION OF ARTHRITIS OF THE SPINE

As I have often told my patients, "God gave us joints which should last for one hundred years." If arthritis develops in the neck or back before that age it is the result of one of the three causes, injury, a chronic disease or a long term nutritional deficiency.

1. PREVENTION OF INJURY is Number One in importance, particularly with men. I never watch a football game, or think back to my own playing years, without wondering if these young men know that the price they pay to play the game may be painful necks and backs in the years to come from traumatic arthritis and intervertebral joint damage.

Repeated heavy lifting is another hazard. Men were never intended to be "beasts of burden." I have never seen the x-rays of a longshoreman's, coal miner's or furniture mover's back who is in his forties or fifties who did not show extensive arthritic changes in the dorso-lumbar vertebrae.

If every package, box, sack or crate, which now must be lifted by one man alone, were limited to not more than 40 pounds - then doctors would see fewer men with degenerative changes in their spines from this type of repeated trauma.

Slips and falls, automobile accidents, ski injuries, high jumps and diving injuries produce most sprains and fractures which result later in a special form of arthritis, named TRAUMATIC ARTHRITIS. It is really a premature form of degenerative disease. One hundred years ago falls from horses caused the most back injuries. Now the doctors see sprains, partial dislocations, and intervertebral disc protrusions and degenerations from work, play and travel accidents. What can a doctor say? "BE MORE CAREFUL."

2. PREVENTION AND EARLY TREATMENT OF INFECTIONS is Number Two in avoiding arthritis, not only in the spine but in any of the joints of the body. "Foci of Infection" as a cause of arthritis is hardly mentioned in recent medical books and journals. Dr. Amos Balkins, who was associated with our clinic, wrote a classic book, "Adventures in Cures." He describes recoveries from arthritis, multiple joint pains and bursitis after finding and treating or removing bad teeth, broken dental roots, jaw abscesses, infected tonsils, chronic sinusitis, inflamed gall bladders, prostates, appendicies and inflammatory pelvic disorders.

A search for such conditions followed by appropriate treatment should be one of the first goals of the physician when a patient is accepted for examination and care.

This book does not have to relate the "horror stories" of patients who were placed on cortisone or some other suppressive drug when removal or treatment of the source of the infection would have prevented or cured the disease.

3. NUTRITIONAL DEFICIENCY is Number Three in the origin of arthritis in the spine. This is particularly true in women and after the child bearing age. Diet fads and weight reducing programs have contributed their toll - as women have avoided milk and dairy products because of the small amount of fat they contain - and thereby developed a CALCIUM DEFICIENCY, which with a LACK OF VITAMIN D produced OSTEOPOROSIS, a softening of the bone of the spine. This results in a shrinking in size and shape of the vertebra, a loss in height of the patient, a stooped posture with the head and neck forward and a dorsal round back deformity. In many cases this leads to compression fractures of the spine, severe pain, and

nerve and spinal cord damage. It is treatable and preventable with the administration of calcium, vitamin D, and a high protein diet.

Frequently a female hormone supplement is prescribed.

C. MANIPULATION OF THE SPINE

By Mr. Lancelot H. F. Walton, M.B., F.R.C.S.
Orthopedic surgeon, Alderney, England

The most common site of back pain is in the lower back, the lumbo-sacral region, although pain often arises from higher up, most commonly in the dorso-lumbar region. This can be determined by the doctor by palpation of the tender areas with gentle pressure, working gradually up the spine. Degenerative changes in the vertebrae and intervertebral discs are logical later in life as these two areas are most subject to strains and injuries. Compression fracture of the 12th thoracic vertebra is frequently missed on x-rays taken for the lumbar spine. Secondary arthritic changes then occur, a cause of severe pain and disability.

Many of my patients with back pain appear to have no disc involvement at all but rather in association with degenerative arthritis of the spine. These changes frequently date back to injuries which occurred many years before, usually during their teens or early twenties.

It is not the x-ray changes seen in the vertebrae, the hypertropic lipping, spurs or sclerosis, but the poor circulation of the attached soft tissues, muscles, fascia, and ligaments which cause the low back pain. The old injuries caused damage to the blood vessels supplying these tissue. Tightness, stiffness and limited motion of the muscles and joints result. When these conditions are treated by gentle manipulation the pain is relieved — but the x-ray changes in the spine appear unchanged.

The purpose of manipulation of the spine by a physician or physical therapist is to secure better motion in the joints, relieve stiffness and improved function of the muscles and ligaments. This is also called "mobilization." It must be done gently, not to cause increased pain, repeatedly, until the improved function become permanent, and skillfully, by persons who have had special training and experience.

In severely painful cases, where even gentle manipulation cannot be tolerated, the treatment is best performed in a hospital under a short general anesthetic.

D. ANKYLOSING SPONDOLYTIS

This is a rare form of spinal arthritis, almost invariably found in males, usually beginning in the teens or twenties. Some cases are linked with rheumatoid disease of the vertebrae, which become inflamed and painful at the onset. Then stiffness follows with a fusion of the vertebrae giving the x-ray appearance of a "bamboo spine". It can occur after chronic infections, such as venereal disease, and Russian doctors have reported cases occurring after acute and poorly treated cases of malaria. In our experience several cases have made remissions or a "complete and permanent relief of symptoms" from the use of Esterene and from anti-protozoal medications.

E. ACUPUNCTURE

DR. PEDRO CHAN, PHD, CA

Acupuncture can be expected to give relief of pain in 80% of patients where that is the chief complaint. Five percent may get a mild recurrence. Ten percent may not be helped because of surgical scars or they may need surgical treatment for their condition.

Several things may interfere with acupuncture treatment. Among these are SOUR FOODS— especially lemon, pineapple, vinegar—ALCOHOL, DRUGS, (except ASPIRIN, which will potentiate acupuncture), SPICED FOODS, SMOKING and OLD SURGICAL SCARS, and OLD INJURY SCARS, such as from wounds or burns.

Acupuncture should be tried three times before deciding that it does not help the patient. If it does not work for some patients there may be a condition present that may require surgical treatment and an M. D. should be consulted accordingly. But, whatever the cause, acupuncture does not make the patient worse in any way.

Chinese medicine developed acupuncture thousands of years ago. The forces of pain travel in "meridians" along which are "acupuncture points". For proper treatment these must be known and located very acccurately for insertion of the needles, which are then twirled, heated, or connected with very low electrical currents. *Acupressure* in some conditions, such as headaches, may be just as effective over the acupressure points.

When surgical scars are present, both external and internal, there is only a fifty percent chance of relief. "Any surgery" in the pain area is a problem for it interferes with the flow of body forces over the meridians. The scars of laminectomy operations are probably the worse. "C" section scars are also difficult sites of pain and interfere with treatments.

When scars are present your doctor may give you relief by injecting the nerves under the scars with water, local anesthetics or other chemical treatment. This may be done by M. D. acupuncturists. Laser irradiation of painful areas and scars may also be indicated and helpful.

For headaches, for example, injection of a point two inches below the umbilicus on the abdomen, or acupuncture at this site, may often bring complete relief. "I never say that acupuncture is a CURE, but I do say that in many cases it will bring PERMANENT RELIEF."

The use of some drugs may mask or prevent the beneficial effects of acupuncture stimulation, particularly the corticosteroids and the NSAIDSs.

Because of this, while I never tell patients to stop taking drugs which have been prescribed by physicians, I give them Chinese GINSING to take for about two weeks before their first acupuncture treatment. Many persons seem to recover on this alone and never need the acupuncture.

I do not believe in prolonged acupuncture therapy. If six to twelve treatments do not give the patient substantial relief, or if they fail to continue to improve after this course of treatment, then the acupuncture treatments should be stopped. The problem with drugs is suppression of the functions of the pituitary gland. Ginsing seems to stimulate some of the functions of this gland, help metabolism, increase body energy and sex functions. Many patients find that they must take it in the mornings or they will be restless at night.

Other patients who may not do well on acupuncture are those that are "too nervous and are afraid of needles". These may not respond well for the first two or three treatments.

Some of the other conditions which respond to acupuncture are:
Chronic pain, neuritis, neuralgia
Headache
Trigeminal neuralgia
Tempero-mandibular syndrome
Low back pain
Menstrual pain
Overweight, for appetite control
Drug and alcohol addiction - especially in group
    therapy
Tinnitis and functional hearing loss
Migraine
Arthritis pain

Patient Procedures:

Questions to ask patients:
Symptoms
Medical History
Any surgery
Drugs the past two weeks
Diet history
Tensions
Sex life

A good patient is one who is relaxed and comfortable. Sit in chair, straight, hips and knees at 90 °. Knees not crossed. Hands on thighs. Massage the neck and shoulders to relax the patient. Say, "If I hurt you, say so."

With ACUPRESSURE use strong pressure, back and forth. Generate a sensation. Producing pain is not acupressure. When the patient says, "I don't feel anything", or says, "I feel it all over", then you are obtaining a response.

In emergency situations when faced with an unconscious patient exert acupressure by pressing very hard with a knuckle at the base of the nose.

(Discussion: After training in Chinese acupuncture in Hawaii in 1977 I have tried it with some success in cases of joint pain due to osteoarthritis. It does relieve some pain. It does not influence the cause or the course of the disease. Now I have learned that the treatment of Dr. Paul K. Pybus of South Africa effects relief of osteoarthritis pain by injecting dilute solutions of a local anesthetic and corticosteriods into these same "trigger points". After seeing his data and demostrations I believe this is the preferred therapy. The method is described in the second edition of RHEUMATOID DISEASE CURED AT LAST. See the bibliography for the reference. R.B.)

Table 19

THE SURGICAL TREATMENT OF ARTHRITIS

Surgical operations for arthritis are not "last resort procedures". They restore joint function and relieve pain.

Minor Office Technics

Joint aspirations of excess synovial fluid
Injections of local anesthetic solutions
Injection of cortico-steroids
Excisions of small cysts, bursae, nodules, exostoses
Corrections of small joint deformities of fingers and
    toes

Hospital Technics

Synovectomy
Correction of major deformities of fingers and toes
Tendon operations
Cervical and Lumbar spine fusions and disectomies
Biopsies for tissue diagnoses
Joint Implants:
    Silastic — Fingers and Toes
    Metal and Plastic — Elbows, Shoulders,
      Hips, Knees, Ankles

Plastic surgery of deformities

GOOD PRE-OPERATIVE CARE IS INSURANCE
FOR GOOD RESULTS

CHAPTER 19

THE SURGICAL TREATMENT OF ARTHRITIS

"It is never too late to start treatment for arthritis." This is the message which every patient with rheumatoid disease or osteoarthritis should receive. Some patients become discouraged when years of treatment and numerous drugs have failed to cure or control the gradual worsening of their illness and disabilities. Others have been told, "Take this medicine and learn to live with your disease." No one has ever told these sufferers that diet, vitamins, exercise, physical therapy and improving their general health would have any effect on their arthritis.

Similarly, many patients develop ugly and physically handicapping deformities of their hands and feet, limitation of their activities by swollen and stiff knees and hips, not realizing that no matter how severe these joints have been damaged there is a method to restore their function and relieve joint pain by modern surgical treatments.

It is important to emphasize here that surgery often can be prevented by a combination of modern medical treatments and use of all of the "fight back" techniques mentioned in this book.

It has been our experience that surgery for arthritis is safer and more successful when the patient has been prepared for the operation by two or three weeks of intensive emphasis on therapy to build up the health and the physical reserves of the body as much as possible.

Within the next year some 30,000 patients in the United States will be told, "We have done everything that is possible with medical treatment for your arthritis. But you have one or more joints that do not respond to conservative treatment. These show by clinical examination and x-rays extensive joint damage from the arthritis. Surigical replacement of the surfaces of these joints is medically indicated and necessary to restore useful and less painful joint function."

If you are one of the patients who has been informed of this recommendation and prognosis, what will be your reaction?

The orthopedic surgeon who has reached this opinion has made a careful study of your case, the severity of the disease, the type of medical treatment you have had, the physical findings in range of motion, pain, swelling, muscle weakness, and by clinical examination for "crepitus" — which is the rubbing of rough joint surfaces together and the x-ray appearance of a loss of cartilage in the joint or joints involved so that he knows that there is no possiblility of natural healing and normal tissue repair. He knows that the cartilage surfaces of joints, once destroyed do not regenerate.

Normal hyalin cartilage, with which the articular surfaces are covered, should last a healthy person "more than 100 years". If this is destroyed by infections within the joint, or suffers a loss of circulation and normal metabolism from inflammation or degeneration which interferes with its blood supply, then the cartilage is gradually dissolved and absorbed and these cartilage cells are replaced with scar tissue which may later become calcified.

Some joints can be allowed to stiffen up naturally, without surgery, as long as they are not painful or are in a location that does not require active motion. These articulations include the spine and sacroiliac joints, the distal or "end" joints in the fingers and toes, the small multiple joints of the wrist, the joints between the heel and the ankle, and the joints in the arch of the foot.

But there are many other joints in the body which do become chronically disabled by pain and joint stiffness. These include the temporal-mandibular articulations of the jaw, the shoulders, elbows, and the metacarpal joints. When their surfaces are severely damaged or destroyed, orthopedic reconstruction surgery can supply satisfactory surface replacements. Preservation of the range of motion in these joints is important because they interfere with the daily physical activities of walking, sitting, riding in a car, normal occupations and employment, and the chores of self-care.

A. DO YOU NEED A JOINT OPERATION?

In rheumatoid arthritis a type of operation called synovectomy may be indicated and necessary in the early stages of the disease, when it has been present for six months to a year or more and is becoming progressively worse in spite of conservative medical treatment. This is particularly true if one or more joints remain chronically swollen, continually painful, limited in motion, or are developing deformitites and the x-rays show beginning of joint space narrowing. The synovectomy actually removes all visible evidences of arthritis in the joint, the inflamed, thickened and damaged joint lining. In some cases this may cause an arrest or remission of the active arthritis in that particular joint or it will delay for several years the necessity for a joint surface replacement.

A synovectomy will require approximately five to ten days of hospital care followed by several weeks of post-operative treatment, during which time the patient will be ambulatory on crutches and follow a course of physical therapy. A synovectomy results in some decrease in motion of the operated joint, but the elimination of pain, swelling, stiffness and a lessening of the process of joint destruction makes this type of operation a worthwhile procedure for many patients.

B. JOINT IMPLANTS

When the loss of joint space by x-ray, which indicates a loss of joint cartilage, has become extensive or complete, then a replacement of these surfaces with a metal and plastic implant fastened to the bone with bone cement will probably be recommended by your orthopedic consultant. During the operation the active arthritis remaining in the joint is removed as in the synovectomy, the necrotic cartilage and bone is excised and the bone surfaces are reshaped and fashioned to take two replacements, one of a non-corroding or a non-rusting metal alloy, the other of an inert high-density polyethyline plastic, and each is fastened to the bone surfaces with methylmethacrylate bone cement.

Your stay in the hospital would probably be from 10 to 16 days, and in lower extremity operations you will be using crutches for from 6 to 12 weeks while you follow a physical therapy and exercise program. In the smaller joints, if more than one implant is necessary several may be done under one anesthetic. The larger joints can be operated a week or so apart, so that the patient seldom is confined to bed for more than two or three days at a time.

These new types of joint implants stand the wear and tear of normal physcial activity very well. The patients may walk, swim, ride bicycles, play golf, drive an automobile and engage in light physical activity and occupations. The average life of the plastic portion of a joint is estimated at 10 to 20 years, when it may be replaced if sufficient wear makes this necessary. The metal portion of the joint should last as long as the patient's life.

C. PREPARATIONS FOR JOINT OPERATIONS

It has been our observation, after performing over 1,000 of these operations in the past five years, that patients who are healthy and well nourished have the easiest courses in the hospital and the best clinical results. Patients who are extremely overweight, or underweight, or who are debilitated by poor nutrition and muscle weakness have a more difficult time.

Before surgery is performed the patient should do the following:
1. Follow a high protein, high vitamin diet.
2. Avoid refined and processed foods.
3. Take therapeutic quantities of vitamin and mineral supplements.
4. Start a program of regular exercises, particularly for the joints which are to be operated.
5. Continue this regimen until your physician determines that you are in good pre-operative condition.

Contrary to the usual opinion, regular exercise does not make arthritis worse. If exercise seems to make the involved joints more painful, limit the amount of exercise to that which produces only slight pain. The discomfort after the proper amount of exercise should not last more than one day.

D. THE RISKS OF AN OPERATION

For the health and welfare of the patients, all of these operations, even the small joints of the fingers and toes, should be done in the hospital to prevent infection and to afford the patient the best nursing and post-operative care. Surveys have shown that in the hospitals where there are special facilities and where a large number of these operations are done the results are better and complications fewer than in hospitals where the operations are performed only occasionally. It is also true that surgeons who are specially trained and perform more of these operations have a higher success rate than surgeons who perform them only occasionally.

In the hospital the patient has a thorough examination by a specialist in general or internal medicine. If the patient is found to have heart and lungs which will withstand an anesthetic well, then there is no problem in the patient being able to undergo the orthopedic operation. There is always some risk in any anesthetic or surgical procedure. But in choosing to do one of these elective operations, we must also consider that the risk is less than the immediate certainty of continued pain and increasing disability. Statistical surveys show that the numbers of complications vary from one half of one per cent up to five per cent in some series. These can be quickly recognized and treated with modern medical techniques.

I frequently use this as an illustration: if a person wishes to travel to a large city he will usually have to ride in an automobile and on the freeways. You know that accidents can occur when you are driving or riding but the statistics on serious accidents are very low. However, if you want to go to the city you assume that risk. The same applies to an elective operation. If you want a good result you must take that small chance and risk of a complication which may prolong your treatment. In medicine we call this the "risk vs. benefit factor". This must be considered carefully by every patient and the physician. Referring to my own experience, some of the first combined plastic and metal joint implants were performed more than 20 years ago. These patients are still walking with these artificial joint surfaces and live useful and comfortable lives. The introduction of bone cement, in the past ten years, has made these implants stronger and more effective. Their manufacture in England has been equaled or exceeded in quality by those made in the United States. Instruments and techniques have been improved and these operations are safe and practicable.

E. TYPES OF JOINT IMPLANTS
HANDS AND FEET

Flexible joints made from silicone rubber can be successfully used to replace stiff joints in the fingers and toes. The material is elastic. When the stiff joint is removed by surgery, the implant is inserted into a space between the bones of the fingers or toes to permit a good range of motion without pain. They are made in sizes for all fingers and toes and have been in use and improved for many years. Usually one hand is done at a time, so the patient will have the other hand for eating, dressing, and self care.

The smaller distal joints of the thumb, fingers, and toes are more frequentlly "arthrodesed:" fused or made stiff in a normal functional position. A very small joint is usually more useful if it is stiff than if it is flexible but weak.

In the feet, removal of the deformed joint is often all that is necessary, because toes do not bear any significant weight. Toe deformities can be corrected, and bunions and exostoses removed, without using joint implants.

In the wrist, the surgeon has a choice of either a movable prosthesis or a fusion operation. For people who need to use their wrists for heavy physical activities, a fusion is better. Those who need their wrist for flexibility prefer the implants.

ELBOWS

Two or three types of implants are available for replacement of stiff or very painful elbows. They consist of two parts, one of metal and the other of plastic, fastened together with a hinge. This gives the patient a full range of useful motion. The implants are fastened to the humerus (arm bone) and the ulna (forearm bone) with plastic bone cement.

SHOULDERS

There are two types of shoulder implants: "restrained" and "unrestrained." The restrained implant has a hinge, making it strong but somewhat limited in motion. The unrestrained implant is held together with the patient's own muscles and ligaments. It has good range of motion without pain but is only as strong as the patient's own muscles. The advantage of a shoulder implant is freedom of motion without pain in a joint that is very necessary for almost all daily body activities.

SPINE

Diseased or deformed joints of the cervical spine and lumbar spine are most often treated by a spinal fusion, usually with a bone graft taken from a part of the pelvis. This gives the patient a strong neck or back and relieves the joint weakness and the pain.

HIPS

"Total hips" have had the longest history of successful surgical operations and are probably the most useful of all joint implants. I first operated and inserted hip implants of metal and plastic in patients who have been using them for over 20 years. These early operations are still without pain and have a very useful range of motion.

The average wear of a hip, knee, or ankle implant is from 10 to 20 years and varies with the body weight of the patient. After that time, the plastic portion may need replacement. The metal part of the implant will last the life of the patient.

There are two types of hip implants: "Double cup," where a plastic cup is inserted in the pelvis and a metal cup is used over the head of the femur; or "total hip," where the neck of the femur is replaced with a metal stem which goes down the shaft of the femur. These come in many types, and the orthopedic surgeon usually chooses the one with which he has had the most training and the best experience. The best of these originally came from England or Germany; now they have been duplicated or improved in this country, and the American made joint implants are very high in quality and are giving excellent service. Recently, we have done *bilateral* hip implants in two patients, and both are now walking 2 to 4 miles a day without pain.

ANKLE

Ankle implants are used where walking and standing on the ankle is painful and the joint shows extensive deterioration. The fused ankle or stiff ankle is completely free of pain. An ankle implant is not entirely pain-free, but the degree of pain is greatly reduced. Weight is borne on a small area. For this reason the success rate in ankle implants has not been as great as in other joints.

KNEES

The knee joint operations are among the most difficult, requiring a high degree of skill and experience from the orthopedic surgeon. Statistics show that hospitals which do a larger number of knee implants have a greater percentage of success than hospitals where very few are performed. The knee implant must be individualized for each patient and each knee. Among the 20 to 30 types offered by various manufacturers, the surgeon must pick the one which suits the patient's case the best. We have found that the *Marmor prosthesis* is the best for single compartment arthroplasties, where only half the joint needs to be replaced; the *Townley implant* is used when the entire joint surface and the kneecap need to be recovered.

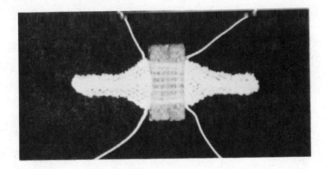

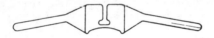

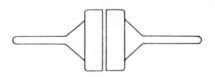

FINGER IMPLANT

HIP IMPLANT

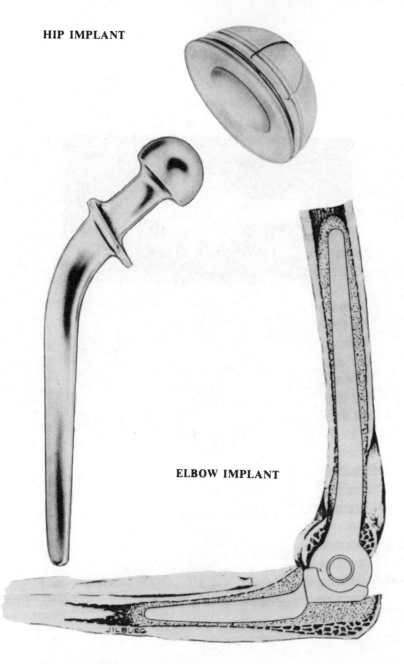

ELBOW IMPLANT

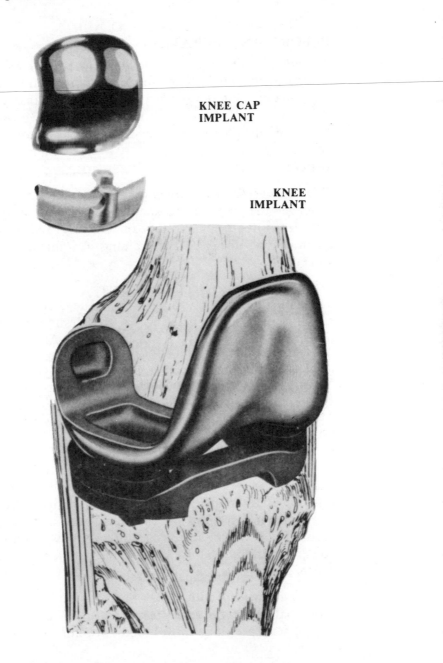

**KNEE CAP
IMPLANT**

**KNEE
IMPLANT**

F. QUESTIONS YOU SHOULD ASK
BEFORE AN OPERATION

In what hospital will the operation be performed?
Your surgery should be performed in a hospital which does many joint replacement operations so that the technicians in the operating room, the nurses on the floor, and the physical therapy technicians are familiar with the special routines necessary for the joint implant patient.

Who will perform the operation?
Whoever the surgeon, he should be certified by the American Board of Orthopedic Surgery and have taken special post-graduate training in joint implant surgery.

What kind of anesthetic will I have?
These operations can be done either under a general or spinal anesthesia, depending on the desires of the patient and his general physical condition. Anesthesia is not a "deep" or heavy anesthetic; patients for this surgery have very few respiratory complications.

What kind of surgical implant will be used?
There are some 100 different joint implants now being used: 30 for the hip, 20 for the knee, and 50 for the neck, shoulders, wrists, elbows, fingers, and feet. The use of metal and plastic implants and bone cement to take the place of the diseased joints has some risk, but probably less than a tenth of the dangers you encounter in traveling on the freeways. In a good hospital you will be in the care of people who know how to prevent and treat any emergency situation which might arise.

How much will it cost?
Most patients who have insurance or one of the government programs have good *hospital* insurance

coverage. The surgeon's fee may be considerably higher than the surgical allowance from the insurance carrier. The total fees should be known and discussed before you go to the hospital so you will not have unpleasant surprises when the bills come in from the surgeon, the assisting surgeon, the consulting internist, the anesthesiologist, and sometimes from other opooialists.

Will I be on a special diet?
Ask your physician whether you may continue on your nutritional diet while in the hospital. Will you be able to take your own, or will he prescribe vitamin and mineral supplements from the hospital pharmacy?

Will the operating room be specially designed for orthopedic surgery?
The operation should be performed in a room where the air is especially clean and filtered to make it more safe for orthopedic operation, particularly joint implants.

Will antibiotics be used?
Ask your surgeon if he uses antibiotics, perferably as a local solution to irrigate the surgical wound during the operation and after. Does he also give antibiotics systemically to prevent infections and complications?

Will special precautions be taken to prevent blood clots?
To prevent thrombophlebitis and embolisms, or "blood clots," intravenous solutions such as Dextran and heparin are often given to thin the blood and prevent excessive clotting in the vein. Intermittent positive pressure cuffs on the legs are frequently used after surgery on the thighs and legs until the patient's own muscles can resume active exercise at frequent times during the day.

Table 20

THE HOME TREATMENT OF ARTHRITIS

Putting It All Together

CHECK LIST: **DATE:**
1. Select your personal physician   _____
2. History and physical examination   _____
3. X-ray and laboratory tests   _____
4. Medical and arthritis diagnoses made _____
5. Dietary and Hair analyses completed _____
6. Consultation, if necessary   _____
7. Medical treatment started, Medicines _____
8. Nutritional program began   _____
9. Plan of rest and exercise   _____
10. Arthritis Vaccine   _____
11. Yucca food supplements   _____
12. Vitamin and mineral supplements   _____
13. Hot therapeutic baths daily   _____
14. Supervised physical therapy   _____
15. Avoiding nightshade foods   _____
16. Avoiding alcohol and nicotine   _____
17. Modified work or employment   _____
18. Filing for disability insurance   _____
19. Getting family and friends to
        cooperate in the program   _____
20. Dates of your follow-up visits
        to the doctor   _____

CHAPTER 20

THE HOME TREATMENT OF ARTHRITIS
PUTTING IT ALL TOGETHER

ARTHRITIS IS NOT A HOSPITAL TREATED DISEASE, except rarely in an acute onset and for arthritis surgery. It is a condition to be treated in the patient's home, with the full knowledge by the patient of the diagnosis, the necessary treatment and the cooperation of the patient's family. The doctor does his part with examination, ordering laboratory tests, requesting x-rays and prescribing any appropriate medicines. The patient fills the prescriptions at the drug store, takes the medicine home, then the actual treatment begins. It is the beginning of another way of life. The patient must FIGHT BACK AGAINST ARTHRITIS.

EVERY DAY THERE ARE DECISIONS TO BE MADE:

Rest—*How many hours a day?*
Work—*Can the present occupation be continued?*
Diet—*What changes should be made?*
Vitamins—*Which ones to take and how many?*
Medicines—*Are they going to do the job?*
The Future—*Recovery, or further disability?*
Time—*Weeks, months, years, or a lifetime?*

A HOME TREATMENT ROUTINE

A typical regime consists of three parts, medical, nutritional and home physical therapy.

1. MEDICATIONS prescribed by your physician. These should be reduced as your symptoms and signs gradually subside. Don't become "addicted" to medicines, for pain, for sleep, or for relief of inflammation. Make regular visits to your physician

but have him prescribe the most mild and safe drugs your condition will permit.

2. NUTRITIONAL PROGRAMS include natural and fresh foods whenever possible, vitamin and mineral supplements, and a herbal extract such as yucca is recommended. Avoid foods which are excessively processed, contain artificial preservatives and additives, or which are high in sugar, starch or fat. Avoid the nightshade foods, tobacco and alcoholic beverages, excess tea and coffee.

3. DAILY HOT BATHS and exercises are the absolutely necessary elements of home physical therapy. A full range of motion for every joint in the body should be attempted every day. Sister Elizabeth Kenny discovered in treating poliomyelitis that each exercise should be done three times twice a day to keep the joints and muscles as flexible as possible.

Then, each exercise should be done against some resistance, isometrics or with weights or springs. They should be done until you begin to feel tired or in a little pain. As Richard Simmons says of exercises, "If it doesn't hurt, it doesn't help". That is also true with arthritis.

Walking, swimming and bicycling are the preferred activities for those who can participate. Walking two miles a day, three or four times a week will keep you in good condition. When swimming or bicycling continue until you feel tired or "get out of breath". Then rest, then try again, twice more.

The contraction and relaxation of muscles act as pumps for the blood, increasing the flow into the joints, bringing oxygen and nourishment and taking away the by-products of metabolism and disease.

Deep hot baths are the best forms of heat for arthritis. Pools or spas are better than bath tubs because of more uniform heat. The best temperatures are from 102° to 104°, for five to ten minutes, repeated three times with cooling off periods in between baths.

Small paraffin baths may be purchased for home use for patients with severe involvement of both hands.

Practical Ways Of
COPING WITH YOUR
ARTHRITIS

Has arthritis limited the motion of some of your joints so that it interferes with your work or leisure activities? Is it difficult or impossible to perform essential personal tasks such as feeding yourself, dressing, or grooming?

There are a number of ways to modify your home and work surroundings to be more functional and increase your independence. You may need to reorganize, simplify, or even eliminate some of your routine daily activites. If you have difficulty walking, slippery floors are particularly hazardous. Throw rugs and anything that might be tripped over should be removed. Steps and long corridors should be equipped with handrails.

WORK HABITS

It is important to simplify household tasks to avoid stress, strain, and fatigue whenever possible. Organizing "work centers," where all items for specific jobs are kept within each reach, can save much wasted motion. For example, set up your ironing area so you can reach for a moistened article of clothing, iron it, and then hang it on an adjacent stand while remaining seated. Your kitchen can be arranged so that your work progresses from refrigerator to counter top to stove—with the fewest unnecessary steps possible.

Certain household tasks provide excellent opportunities for useful exercise. Use large circular motions while dusting to give you valuable shoulder motion. Ironing with long strokes and your arm kept straight provides the same motion. When vacuuming, make long forward thrusts and then pull the vacuum or hose handle back close to your body—extending, flexing, and exercising your arm. The same kind of stroke should be used in mopping floors.

THE BATHROOM

If you have difficulty getting on and off the toilet, a raised seat can be used. Grab bars near the toilet also can help. Position grab bars near the bathtub or shower to aid you in getting in and out safely. A low chair or stool with rubber leg tips in the tup can help you get into and out of the bathtub and bathe without help. A rubber suction mat on the floor of the tub is a good precaution against slipping. If your hands are weak, you may want to install long-handled faucets on the sinks in both the bathroom and kitchen.

FURNITURE

Some changes in your furniture may be necessary, especially if you have deformities that are permanent. If pain and weakness make it difficult to get up from a low chair or bed, putting unnecessary strain on damaged joints, your bed or chair should be higher than normal and fairly firm. A simple way to raise a chair or bed is to put wood blocks under the legs. If you sit on a stool, it should provide support for your back. Electric or hydraulic powered "lift" chairs are available that raise you at a touch of a button to a standing position.

LIVING WITH A WHEELCHAIR

If you are confined to a wheelchair, moving around in your home can create special problems. Halls and rooms must be large enough to allow the wheelchair to turn, and doorways must be wide enough to permit the chair to pass through. Door thresholds may need to be removed; steps can sometimes be replaced with a gradually sloping ramp.

Light switches and electrical outlets should be located at a height convenient to reach from the wheelchair. Switches and other controls on appliances may need to be modified, or a piece of adaptive equipment provided, so you can reach and operate the controls.

Additional leg space under counters, tables, and desks may be necessary. Kitchen cabinets equipped with a pull-out work counter or dropleaf work surface are an excellent solution. A wheelchair tray may provide an adequate substitute for a work counter. Folding or sliding closet doors are more practical than doors with hinges.

SELF-HELP DEVICES

A variety of simple self-help devices available commercially can also make your life easier. Such energy-savers as electric can openers, jar openers, long-handled shoehorns, telephone holders and dialers can usually be found in department or hardware stores, novelty shops, or by mail order. With a little ingenuity, you can design your own specialty items or make simple adaptions to existing implements and tools to suit your specific needs.

The following suggestions should give you ideas for other self-help aids to buy, adapt, or design:

WIRE BASKET

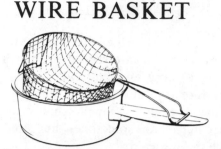

COOKING When cooking foods in water or oil, a wire basket can save the effort of lifting the pan when full to strain the food and avoid dangerous spills. A soap holder under the mixing bowl will hold it securely. Use lightweight plastic containers and foil for storing food in the refrigerator. Aluminum cookware is lighter than stainless steel or ironware.

EATING UTENSILS If you have a problem with your grip, look for eating utensils with built-up or extra-long handles—or adapt existing ones to suit your needs. "Selectagrip" cutlery is designed for those with grip problems and includes a "splayed" (a knife, fork, and spoon all in one) and a sipping spoon, as well as a hand strap and oversized plastic handles in three designs.

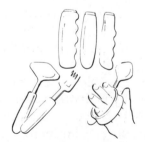

'SELECTAGRIP' CUTLERY

CLEANING A simple to make footmop will save a lot of bending. A long handled dustpan is easy to make if you can't find one in the store.

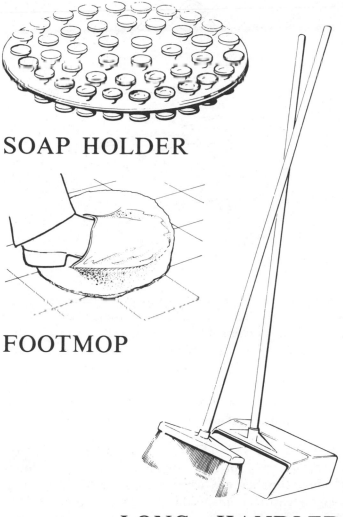

SOAP HOLDER

FOOTMOP

LONG—HANDLED DUSTPAN

RETRIEVING STICKS

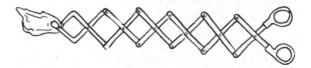

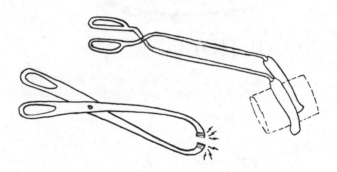

REACHING Long-handled retrievers are available in a variety of sizes and designs—tongs, scissors, or expandible pinchers. Or you can make your own with a stick and a clothespin. These very useful devices will save you much stretching, stooping, climbing, and straining for out-of-reach items. They can also hold a sponge or dust rag; those fitted with a magnetic tip can pick up pins, needles, etc.

MOVING HEAVY ITEMS A cart or small table on casters is handy for transporting laundry, dishes, food, cleaning supplies, etc. while putting less of a burden on weight-bearing joints. You may have to replace door thresholds with flat metal strips so it will easily move from room to room. Don't lift heavy things if you can push or roll them instead.

ELECTRICAL PLUG WITH HANDLE

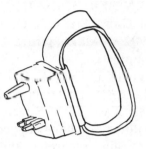

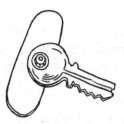

LARGE HANDLED DOORKEY

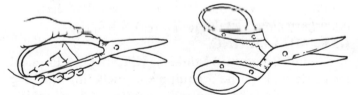

LONG-HANDLED SCISSORS AND TONGS

MISC. ITEMS A large handle for your door key can be made by bolting on a square or T-shaped piece of wood or metal. An electric plug with a handle can make it easier to insert and pull out of the socket. Long-handled scissors, tongs, and other tools are available commercially.

Self-Help Devices Source List

SHELTERED WORKSHOP AND REHABILITATION SERVICES, INC.
200 Court Street, P.O. Box 310, Binghamton, N.Y. 13902 • Manufacture "U-shaped" stocking aid. Pamphlets.

VOCATIONAL GUIDANCE & REHABILITATION SERVICES
2289 East 55th Street, Cleveland, Ohio 44103 • Clothing for handicapped women, including dresses, suits, slips, separates, and accessories. A few items for men. Pamphlets.

WINCO PRODUCTS
Winfield Co., In., 3062 46th Avenue, N., St. Petersburg Fla. 33714 • Self-help equipment including raised toilet seats, shower/commode chairs, walkers, safety bars.

FASHION-ABLE, INC.
Rocky Hill, N.J. 08553 • Mail order clothes for the handicapped woman, featuring specially designed undergarments. Catalogue.

G. E. MILLER, INC.
484 South Broadway, Yonkers, N.Y. 10705 • Physical medicine and self-help equipment, including stocking and dressing aids, eating utensils, home-making equipment.

FRED SAMMONS, INC.
Box 32, Brookfield, Ill. 60513 • Self-help aids, including built-up eating utensils, Velcro tape closure, personal hygiene aids, kitchen aids, shoe fasteners and stocking aids.

CLEO LIVING AIDS
3957 Mayfield Rd., Cleveland, Ohio 44121 • Self-help equipment including clothing, eating aids, shower and bath devices. Catalogue.

SEXUAL ACTIVITY AND ARTHRITIS

Will sexual activity make your arthritis worse? At the Moss Rehabilitation Hospital in Philadelphia, research on this very question reveals the following results as reported by Dr. George Ehrlich of Temple University Medical School.

The sex act releases a hormone that acts like cortisone, probably from stimulation of the adrenal glands. This may relieve pain and stiffness in specific parts of the body, such as the muscles and joints, and the beneficial effects may last up to 6 hours. The brain also release hormones (endomorphins) into the blood stream that are also pain-relieving substances.

Any form of exercise—as sexual activity certainly is—improves the circulation of the entire body. It speeds up breathing, the pulse rate, and the rate of circulating blood; it increases oxygen to the muscles and joints; and it improves joint motion and flexibility. All these body functions benefit the arthritis patient.

However, sexual activity may be uncomfortable to some patients, who will seek body positions and sexual activities that are stimulating but not too uncomfortable.

There is no medical evidence of sexual activity causing injury or making arthritis worse. On the contrary, it is on the recommended list of functions for arthritis patients.

GUIDE TO PHYSICAL ACTIVITIES
FOR THE ARTHRITIS PATIENT

Posture

Whether walking, standing, sitting or even sleeping, good posture is important for people with arthritis. Poor posture can make arthritis worse. As for standing, you should stand straight, head high, shoulders back, stomach in, hips and knees straight.

Sitting

Keep good posture when sitting down. Use straight-back armchair with firm seat. Sit with head up, shoulders back, stomach in, feet flat on floor. Use arms of chair to stand up slowly.

Resting/Sleeping

Patients with rheumatoid arthritis should avoid bent knees or arms. Lie straight at sides, knees and hips straight. Put plywood board between mattress and bedspring. NEVER put a pillow under your knee. Use a firm mattress, and if you need a pillow under your head, use a thin one. Keep sheets and blankets loose over your feet, perhaps by using a blanket support. If your arthritis is in your back, you may need a different position for sleeping—ask your physician.

Walking

Walk erect, as in standing position, arms swinging freely at sides, let your weight shift easily from one side to the other. Don't carry heavy packages in one hand. A light-weight shoulder bag is a good idea. If legs or knees are involved, a cane will make walking easier.

Arrange your work so that you are in a comfortable relaxed position. Sit down to work. It's easier to stir a bowl in the sink than high up on the counter.

Don't strain unstable joints such as fingers, elbows, knees or ankles. (Your doctor will discuss this with you.) To protect thumb joints, open milk containers with heels of the hands, rather than with thumbs.

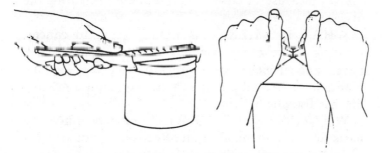

If your hands are affected, avoid old, stressful ways of opening jars, wringing out laundry, etc. Instead use a jar opener and other helpful tools to reduce stress on joints. Use tools with large handles.

Use the palms of your hands for lifting and pushing. Push instead of pulling.

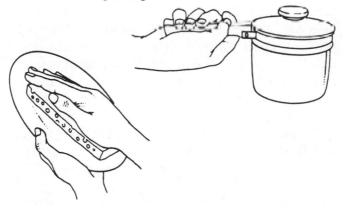

Dishwashing should be done with fingers kept straight as much as possible. If a dishwasher is available use it in preference to washing by hand.

PUTTING IT ALL TOGETHER

There are so many questions and uncertainties in every case of arthritis that the patient should take every known measure of effort and treatment in fighting the disease.

WHAT IS THERE TO LOSE? Next to cancer, arthritis is the most disabling disease a patient can have—and it never causes death, but can become gradually worse all a patient's life, sometimes making life hardly worth living.

WHAT IS THERE TO WIN? Good health is the basis of any enjoyment of life. Recovery from arthritis must be pursued until there is a "permanent relief of symptoms."

WHAT ARE YOUR CHANCES? You may be told that "your arthritis has no known cause and no known cure." Yet the treatments and methods described in this book have produced improvement, remissions and recoveries in from seventy to ninety-four per cent of all patients with all types of arthritis. None of these programs have ever made a patient worse. Twenty-four per cent report that their disease has been arrested but they do not regain full health. Six per cent have some joints that have been so permanently damaged by disease that the deformities must be accepted unless surgical replacement is possible.

Where you will be in this list depends upon what you do. This book is a guide. The rest is up to you.

APPENDIX I

ROBERT BINGHAM, M.D., F.A.C.S.

The author is founder and director of the Desert Arthritis Medical Center and Clinic in Desert Hot Springs, California. Since 1959 this institution has treated many thousands of patients, children and adults with various forms of arthritis, from all parts of the United States and Canada. The emphasis is to restore health to the patient while using innovative and non-injurious methods of treatment, nutrition, exercise and hot mineral water baths.

Doctor Bingham was raised in the medical profession. His father, W. J. Bingham, M. D. was a pioneer medical missionary in Guatemala, Nicaragua and Mexico, and a "horse and buggy doctor" in Colorado, where Robert Bingham was born.

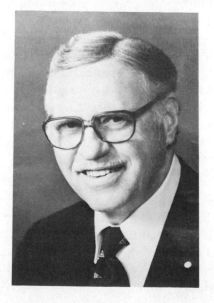

He graduated from the University of Redlands, California and from the School of Medicine of the University of Colorado in Denver. After a two year internship at the Hospital of the University of Pennsylvania in Philadelpia he became a resident at the New York Orthopaedic Hospital and Dispensary and the Columbia Presbyterian Hospital in New York City, with a special interest in crippled children's surgery.

After four years of service as an orthopedic surgeon during World War II, two of which were in the South Pacific, he started practice in Riverside, California. He has been an attending or consulting surgeon in many hospitals in the County of Riverside and was the founding director of the Angel View Crippled Childrens Foundation in Desert Hot Springs, California. During the years of poliomyelitis epidemics he served as chief of the medical staff of the Sister Kenny Poliomyelitis Hospital in El Monte, California. He was assistant clinical professor of orthopedic surgery at the College of Medical Evangelists in Loma Linda, California. He now lives and does his arthritis surgical operations in Orange County where he has been the chairman of the department of surgery at Midwood Commmunity Hospital in Stanton, California.

From the beginning of his medical education and practice he has treated arthritis patients medically and surgically. He was trained in clinical investigation and has been the author of over sixty medical papers, three books and is the editor of the newsletter, ARTHRITIS AND HEALTH NEWS.

He is certified by the American Board of Orthopaedic Surgery, a Fellow of the American College of Surgeons and the American Academy of Orthopaedic Surgery, a member of the Pan-Pacific Surgical Association, the International College of Applied Nutrition, and he has been the editor of the Journal of Applied Nutrition.

His hobbies are sailing, photography and the collecting of old and rare cameras, and his home computer. He is a regent of the University of Redlands, California and the curator emeritus of the California Museum of Photography at the University of California, Riverside.

Some of his contributions to medical knowledge include studies on blood coagulation, the use of local antibiotics to prevent wound infection, a non-adherent surgical gauze, and the use of yucca in the treatment of arthritis. He has collaborated in the use of an arthritis vaccine and was the first doctor in the United States to use and recommend the anti-protozoal drug therapy discovered by the late Dr. Roger Wyburn-Mason for rheumatoid arthritis.

Since the formation of The Roger Wyburn-Mason & Jack M. Blount Foundation for the Eradication of Rheumatoid Disease he has been the chairman of the medical and scientific advisory committee in their program of research on the cause and treatment of rheumatoid arthritis and allied protozoal diseases. (See Appendix III.)

DESERT HOT SPRINGS

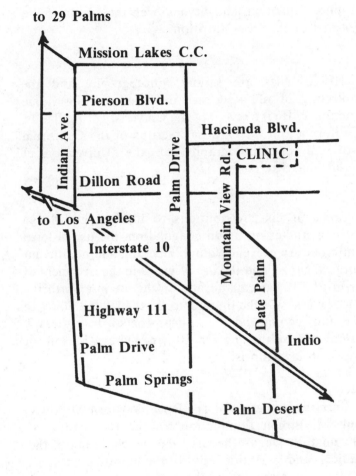

APPENDIX II

THE DESERT ARTHRITIS MEDICAL CLINIC is nationally known for its innovative and conservative treatment of arthritis diseases. Organized in 1967 as a California non-profit community clinic it is sponsored and partially supported by the DESERT ARTHRITIS MEDICAL CENTER, INC., a California charitable and educational foundation for the investigation and treatment of arthritis and allied diseases. Contributions to the Center are tax-exempt under the IRS and the State of California. Some of its projects have been the development of an arthritis vaccine, the use of yucca extract as an herbal food supplement for arthritis patients, the treatment of a group of patients with the Esterene substance and pioneering the use of anti-protozoal drugs for rheumatoid disease. Crippled children are treated without charge, and no patient is refused care because of race, religion, color or ability to pay.

The DESERT HOT SPRINGS MEDICAL CLINICS are a partnership of physicians who supply medical services to the patients and the community of Desert Hot Springs. General medicine, internal medicine, arthritis and orthopedic surgical examinations and treatments are provided at the two clinics. X-ray, laboratory and physical therapy departments are located at the main clinic on Mountain View Road. The Palm Drive Clinic is mostly family practice. Both clinics treat minor medical and surgical emergencies. Consultation services are arranged with a specialist in Palm Springs, only 15 miles away, and in Palm Desert, as are the facilities of the Desert Hospital and the Eisenhower Medical Center. Some patients requiring arthritis surgery go to Midwood Community Hospital in Stanton, Orange

County, not far from Disneyland and Knott's Berry Farm.

A project planned for 1985 is the MOUNTAIN VIEW SPA-HOTEL which will be built adjacent to the clinic for out-of-town patients and guests. The restaurant will offer special menus and foods for arthritis patients and their companions.

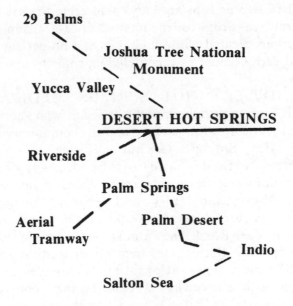

NEARBY SPOTS TO VISIT

APPENDIX III

The ROGER WYBURN-MASON & JACK M. BLOUNT FOUNDATION FOR ERADICATION OF RHEUMATOID DISEASE is also known as "The RHEUMATOID DISEASE FOUNDATION". It was established to support research and treatment into the discoveries by the late Dr. Wyburn-Mason of protozoa as a cause for rheumatoid and some other chronic diseases. Dr. Blount, a physician totally disabled by rheumatoid arthritis, recovered with the use of antiprotozoal drugs and he has treated more than fifteen thousand patients by this method, which he learned from a medical paper in ORTHOPEDIC REVIEW by Dr. Bingham.

The Foundation has published the book, RHEUMATOID DISEASES CURED AT LAST by Anthony diFabio and published and distributed by the non-profit, tax exempt and charitable organization. Write to Rt. 4, Box 137, Franklin, TN. 37064. It is free for a $15.00 tax exempt donation through The Rheumatoid Disease Foundation, P. O. Box 17405, Washington, D. C. 20041 or may be purchased for $9.95 plus $1.00 for packing and mailing ($10.95) from The Rheumatoid Disease Foundation, Rt. 4 Box 137, Franklin, TN, 37064.

The Rheumatoid Disease Foundation also provides a treatment protocol for Rheumatoid and Osteo victims and their physicians, free of charge; and a Physicians' Referral List for those who enquire at the Franklin TN address.

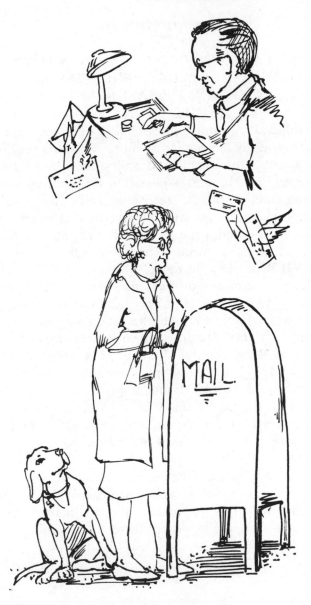

WHEN IN DOUBT —
WRITE A LETTER

APPENDIX IV

LETTERS FROM PATIENTS

This past year we requested letters of recommendations from our patients for a California agency concerned with the quality of medical care. With permission of the patients their letters have been abbreviated for the patients who read this book. They dramatically reveal some of the benefits and results of this arthritis program.

At the Clinic we welcome letters with questions about arthritis or for information about our facilities and treatments. RB

La Porte City, Iowa.
A year after surgery for cancer of the colon, in only one month of time, I developed severe acute rheumatoid arthritis to a degree that made life unlivable.

I obtained *no relief* from all the medicine the Doctors here were able to prescribe.

As my sister had found relief under the care of the Desert Arthritis Medical Clinic — I decided to go to California to try, at least, to see if there was any help for me. With the use of my shoulders and hands in any way I fairly screamed with pain. I had to lie on my back all night. With no one to help me out of bed, and to avoid the use of my hands, I would hook my feet under a window sill to raise my body so I could get out of bed.

After the first week of treatment with arthritis program gave me super relief of pain, stiffness and swelling. In a month I was able to return home in comfort.

In these past five years I have continued to follow the routine that was prescribed for me with no recurrences. KS

Palm Desert, California.
Having severe crippling rheumatoid arthritis for the
past 18 years, I have been in the best hospitals in
California and have seen numerous doctors,
orthopedists and rheumatologists. I was a "hopeless
cripple". I was very ill when I went to the Clinic.

I was started on the "arthritis program". It has help
me to return to a normal life.

I am only a "layman" but I have talked to people, in
fact hundreds, from all parts of the country who have
taken this treatment and feel as I do. Dr. Bingham has
"forgotten more about arthritis than most doctors
know". WLF

Hemet, California.
While staying at a motel in Desert Hot Springs the
manager told us the story of the four year old girl with
crippling arthritis who recovered with the use of the
vaccine therapy and the arthritis treatment program.

She is now free of arthritis, active, beautiful and
extremely grateful.

I have attended lectures at the Clinic and was very
impressed, not only with rheumatoid arthritis but that
help is given crippled children regardless of their
inability to pay for services.

This type of treatment is what suffering arthritic
persons need, and we all know there are thousands
searching for such a remedy other than drugs with
many side effects. SE

Chicago, Illinois.
I have been bothered with arthritis for about 15
years. I have tried several different types of treatment
with several doctors without much success.

I was one of the first patients in the United States to
try the anti-protozoal drugs. Since then, for more than
five years I have been almost free of arthritis pain and

swelling. I wish that there were doctors in this area who would give this treatment. CL

Santa Ana, California.
Our family doctor and one more M. D. said that I "must live with progressing debilitating arthritis". A gloomy prognosis indeed. My husband and I sought another opinion,

We had read of Dr. Robert Bingham's results in several health journals. Thus, when a business associate previously crippled with arthritis told us of his improvement and recommended Dr. Bingham we phoned for an appointment.

After the initial visits and treatment and the anti-protozoal medications, diet, vitamins and mineral my own enthusiasm prompted my husband to join me for an appointment. He is a professional in another field and was impressed with Dr. Bingham's thorough examination, his obvious expertise and success, coupled with his compassionate concern and optimistic manner encouraged us. We had our first hope that with proper attention my arthritic condition would improve.

That hope has been substantiated by the results which followed. His care has provided the blessings of an active functioning wife, mother and grandmother to a very grateful family. SJR

Seal Beach, California.
I have had both rheumatoid arthritis and osteo arthritis for seven years. During this time my rheumatoid disease went into remission after taking Flagyl, although I still take it for a day or two if the disease seems to be coming back.

Due to severe joint damage before taking this medicine Dr. Bingham had to replace one shoulder joint and both knee joints with surgical implants.

In spite of this the treatment has brought me from a wheel chair, to a walker, then a cane, and now I am able to function without any of these. Never has infection set in after such surgery on patients who have taken the anti-protozoal drugs. I have consulted many doctors in the past who cannot provide such successful care. VSA

Laguna Hills, California

My arthritis began in 1959 or 1960. I was a complete wreck from all of the pain and stress I was going through when I first went to the Clinic in 1980. At that time my fingers, legs, toes and feet were all swollen and I had pain in all my joints. I was placed on the Arthritis Program of diet, exercises, vaccine and vitamins for my health and strength.

A year and a half later I was able to walk without a cane and the swelling had gone down in my legs so I was not ashamed to wear a bathing suit for the first time in years. There was just some heat in my left knee, so I know the treatment must be repeated or continued, but I have faith and hope again. TTK

Palm Springs, California.

My husband and I came to the desert area for my health and the treatment of my rheumatoid arthritis. In 1979 my disease had been worsening for several months in spite of cortisone shots I was getting.

By December I could no longer bear the pain throughout my body. I went to the Clinic and had various x-rays and blood tests taken, etc. I also saw a rheumatologist that month who suggested gold, penicillamine or continuing with the steroids.

Dr. Bingham told me that although there was "NO CURE FOR ARTHRITIS" a new approach discovered by Dr. Roger Wyburn-Mason in England offered promise in my type of case. He also described his program which included rest, exercises, nutrition and physical therapy. He advocated the safest and "least harmful" but necessary drugs for treatment.

It was left totally up to me to continue with the rheumatologist or try the Clinic treatment. I decided to "go" with Dr. Bingham's program.

Within two months first taking Flagyl and following the prescribed health routine I found the first improvement in several years. Flexibility of the joints improved. There was less pain. Drugs were stopped except for occasional aspirin. In another four months "I was a new person". My feet had been painful for literally years, and now I could almost forget I had feet. The constant bursitis in my shoulder and arm was gone. My legs, which had felt so heavy I could hardly get up and walk, were "normal" and pain free. Therapy was discontinued and after six months I stopped going to the clinic and drifted off the program.

I know I still have arthritis. My hands bother me now and then. I am a telephone operator and work all day punching keys. But when I start to feel some pain in other joints I get back on my diet. I have not had to take another course of the anti-protozoal medicine, but I'm glad to know it's there if I ever need it again. JV

Torrance, California.
From the latter part of 1981 through the entire year of 1982 I was under the care of my family doctor and a second doctor specializing in arthritis. They diagnosed my problems as rheumatoid arthritis but their medication and treatment did nothing for me. The joints in my arms and legs were becoming more restrictive in their movement.

Early this year I visited Dr. Bingham who also

diagnosed my case as rheumatoid arthritis. After about three or four weeks of his prescribed medication, including the antiprotozoal therapy discovered by Dr. Roger Wyburn-Mason, the movement in the restricted joints increased considerably. My joints have constantly improved since then, and today, except for a few joints, I have regained nearly complete freedom of movement. RVM

Los Angeles, California.
In 1978 I contracted crippling arthritis after a form of what was thought to be a "form of virus". I was treated with drugs "to make me walk again" and other drugs to keep the rheumatoid disease "in remission". But I failed to regain any strength and became fearful of the side effects which were oncoming.

At this point I changed to the Clinic's arthritis program, diet, vitamins, vaccine, hot baths and therapy.

Now I have regained my old vitality and have gone back to work. Occasionally, when weakened by an attack of virus, or overindulgence in work, or worry I realize that my arthritis is still with me. But I know that under the Clinic's guidance I can cope with it, the pain will be gone again, and *I will have no side effects from the treatment.* EL

McFarland California.
In October of 1976, at the age of 48, I developed pains in my shoulders. Joint pains rapidly spread throughout my whole body. I was forced to quit my job as a medical transcriber because I could no longer type or drive a car because of the pain in my fingers and wrists. I became almost totally disabled.

During this time I consulted many doctors. They prescribed aspirin, codeine and other drugs with no relief.

In December I went to a famous medical clinic where I saw a rheumatologist. He admitted me to the hospital where I underwent multiple tests including a bone marrow biopsy. They said they were "looking for leukemia". Finally my condition was diagnosed as "rheumatoid arthritis". I was again given aspirin, which did no good, and codeine, which made me ill. I was told to "Contact other arthritics and learn to live with my problem"!

In 1977 I was reading "NORMA", the autobiography of the famous singer, Norma Zimmer, of the Lawrence Welk Show. She told of her husband's arthritic condition and how after taking Dr. Bingham's treatment he was changed from a helpless cripple to being an avid skiier in a couple of months.

In June of that year I had a check-up and a consultation and started on the arthritic plan to control the protozoal cause of rheumatoid disease and improve my health, hot baths, fasting at first, diet, vaccine and medications. I really appreciated Dr. Bingham's concern with nutrition.

I started to improve very rapidly and in two months resumed my job, started driving, and I have lived normally since that time. I have faithfully continued my treatment and medications when necessary. I am never completely free of pain, but with Dr. Bingham's help and my faith in God I live an absolutely beautiful life. VD

Hemet, California.
My arthritis has been severe for many years. Fortunately my case responded well to the arthritis program and the Flagyl medication. If it wasn't for Dr. Bingham's treatment I probably wouldn't be walking now. So I can't say enough good things for this treatment. ME

Desert Hot Springs.
I live in Desert Hot Springs because the climate and
hot mineral baths are helpful to my arthritis, which I
have had since 1975. When I first became a patient at
the Clinic and started taking Flagyl my rheumatoid
arthritis was so severe that it seemed hopeless I could
ever live a normal, active life again. Due to this
medicine and the Clinic's devotion to return me to
good health I am much improved. I help my husband
in his business, do most of the housework and sing in
the church choir. I can attest that this program at the
Clinic, and wherever it may be available in the United
States, is responsible for my improvement and should
be known by physicians and patients everywhere. ME

Oceanside, California.
I have had a severe case of arthritis since I was 25 years
of age. I am now 71. Until 1978 I had spent most of my
life in northern Ohio, near the Great Lakes of extreme
summer heat and high humidity. Over the many years I
did approach many, many doctors for help. Each one
would say, "There is no help for arthritis." They would
merely suggest that I take aspirin. Some would
recommend a costly form of arthritis tablet, which
seldom seemed to have any effect, whatsoever. When I
was up to 24 aspirin tablets a day I finally realized that
something better was much needed.

On a visit to California I had a consultation with a
medical doctor in Mexico, and I formed the opinion
that I did not want to take his cortisone medicines
either. In ten minutes time, without any physical
examination, and with two x-rays taken over street
clothes, I was told that I was "In a bad state" and
would "need four operations immediately."

Soon after that I was reading in LET'S LIVE
magazine what Dr. Robert Bingham was doing for

patients at the Desert Arthritis Medical Clinic at Desert Hot Springs, California. A telephone call obtained an appointment. After a three hour history and physical examination, the most complete I have ever had over the years, Dr. Bingham related the details of his findings to me and later gave me a written copy for my medical records. He recommended that I discuss this with my family. Then, if interested, make a later appointment to start treatment. I was so "sold" on his evaluation and recommendations that I started treatment that day, the complete arthritis health program.

This was in 1979 and 1980.

After three months all arthritis pain left my body and has never returned. Since the beginning Dr. Bingham has prescribed none of the usual arhtritis medicines, no gold, no cortisone has ever been included. Proper nutrition, vitamins, minerals and physical therapy have all helped.

To this day I feel happy, without pain and extremely healthy. I candidly believe, had I not gotten the help Dr. Bingham gave me, I would not be alive today. PCV

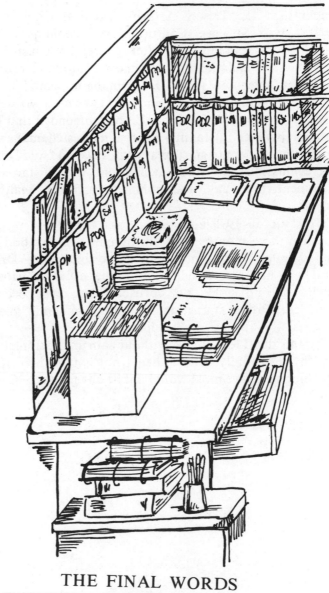

THE FINAL WORDS
ON ARTHRITIS ARE
YET TO BE WRITTEN

APPENDIX V

REFERENCES FOR PATIENTS AND PHYSICIANS

The practice of medicine and the treatment of disease are arts based on science. Until medical science has all or at least more of the answers to the causes and cures for arthritis any treatment which has helped some people should be considered with tolerance and further investigation.

Those who wish to obtain additional information should obtain one or more of the following books. If they are not available on special order from your local book store you may write directly to the publishers or distributors:

RHEUMATOID DISEASES CURED AT LAST
by Anthony di Fabio
> The Rheumatoid Disease Foundation
> Franklin, TN 37064 (615) 646-3757
> ($9.95 + $1.00 postage)
> or for $15.00 Donation:
> The Rheumatoid Disease Foundation
> P.O. Box 17405, Washington, D.C. 20041

NATURAL RELIEF FOR ARTHRITIS
by Carol Keough and the
> Editors of Prevention Magazine
> Rodale Books, Rodale Press, Inc.
> 33 East Minor Street,
> Emmaus, PA 18049 ($15.95)

PATIENT NUTRITION HANDBOOK
> Desert Arthritis Medical Clinic
> 13-630 Mountain View Road
> Desert Hot Springs, CA 92240 ($6.00)

ARTHRITIS
by John L. Decker
    Arthritis Clearing House
    P.O. Box 9782
    Arlington, VA 22209 (Free)

PATIENT INFORMATION BOOKLETS
    The Arthritis Foundation
    1314 Spring St. N.W.
    Atlanta, GA 30309 (Free)

THE CAUSATION OF RHEUMATOID DISEASE
by Roger Wyburn-Mason
    A new Concept in Medicine, a Precis and Addenda
    The Rheumatoid Disease Foundation
    Rt. 4, Box 137 Franklin, TN 37064
    (For a $15.00 donation.)

ARTHRITIS, A COMPREHENSIVE GUIDE
by James F. Fries, M.D.
    Addison-Wesley Publishing Co., Inc.
    Reading, MA 01867 ($9.95)

ARTHRITIS AND HEALTH NEWS
    Arthritis Patients Association
    P.O. Box 730
    Yorba Linda, CA 92686
    (Subscription price $11.00 year)

THE ARTHRITIS HELPBOOK
by Kate Lorig, R.N. and James F. Fries, M.D.
    Addison-Wesley Publishing Co., Inc.
    Reading, MA 01867
    (Paperback $7.95 Hardback $11.95)

BIBLIOGRAPHY

1. Ailkman, Lonnelle: "Yucca, Nature's Healing Arts; from Folk Medicine to Modern Drugs." *National Geographic Magazine,* 157:25, 39, 54, 1977.

2. Allbrecht, W. A.: "Soil Fertility," *J. Acad. Applied Nutrition,* 1: 7-27, 1947.

3. Babb, Richard R. et al: "Arthritis Rounds, Malabsorption." *Arthritis and Rheumatism,* 10:63, Feb. 1967.

4. Bailey, Herbert: "GH-3; Will It Keep You Younger Longer? Procaine." *Bantam Books, New York,* 1977.

5. Balls, Edward K.: "Early Uses of California Plants. Yucca." 44-47, *Univ. of Calif. Press, Berkeley,* 1962.

6. Berkstein, Kanarek, A.: "Vaccine." *Medical Review, Mexico,* 65: 25, May 25, 1962.

7. Bingham, Robert: "Yucca Plant Suponin in the Management of Arthritis." *Journal of Applied Nutrition,* 17:45-51, 1975.

8. Bingham Robert: "New and Effective Approaches in the Prevention and Treatment of Arthritis." *Journal of Nutrition.* 28: 38-47, 1976.

9. Bingham, Robert: "Yucca . .in the Treatment of Hypertension and Hypercholesterolemia." *J. Amer Acad. Applied Nutrition,* 30: 3 & 4, 1978.

10. Bingham, Robert: "Arthritis News Today." *Arthritis and Health News.* Vol. 1-5, No. 1-65, 1978-1983. Arthritis Patients Assn., Yorba Linda, CA.

11. Bonner, J., Varner, J.E.: "Plant Biochemistry; Yucca." 27: 673-715, *Academic Press,* New York 1975.

12. Carter, R.F.: "Amoebic Meningo-encephalitis, Protozoa." *Trans. Royal Soc. Trop. Med. Hyg,* 66: 195-197, 1972.

13. Chang E.S., Owens S.: "Protozoa." *J. Immun.* 92: 313, 1964.

14. Christian, C.L.: "Rheumatoid Arthritis." (in) Immunological Diseases, *Samter, M. ed.* 1015-27. Little Brown, Boston, 1971.

15. Comroe, Bernard I.: "Arthritis and Allied Conditions." *Arthritis Vaccines.* Lea & Febiger, Philadelphia, 1944.

16. Crowe, H.W.: "Vaccine Treatment of Chronic Arthritis." *Oxford University Press,* England, 1932.

17. Cursone, R.T.M.; Brown, T.J.; Keys, E.A.: "Protozoa." *Lancet,* ii: 875.

18. Dobell, C.: "The Amoeba Living in Man." *John Bale, Sons, and Danielson, London,* 1919.

19. Dubois, Rene, J.: "Vaccines." *J. Exper. Med.* 71:249, 1939.

20. Ehrlich, George: "Clinical Pharmacology and Therapeutics." *American Family Practice,* 17:4, 467-68, 1979.

21. Eldridge, A.E.: Tobin, J.O.H.: "Protozoa." *Brit. Med. J.,* I:299, 1976.

22. Ely, L.W.; Reed, A.C.; Wyckoff, H.A.: "The Amoeba as the Cause of the Second Grade Type of Chronic Arthritis." *Calif. State J. Med.,* 20:59, 1922.

23. Engel, Arnold; Burch, Thomas A.: "Chronic Arthritis in the United States." *Arthritis and Rheumatism,* 10:61-62, Feb. 1967.

24. Faust, E.C.; Russell, P.T.; Jung, R.C. (editors): "Clinical Parasitology." *Protozoa.* Lea & Febiger, Phildelphia, 1970.

25. Gentry, Howard S.: "The Agave Family in Sonora. Yucca." *U.S. Dept. Articulture Handbook* • *399,* 154-164, U.S.G. P.O., Washington, 1972.

26. Glynn, L.E.: "The Chronicity of Inflammation and its Significance in Rheumatoid Arthritis." *Protozoa. Ann Rheum. Dis.,* 27: 105-111, 1968.

27. Griffin, LaDean: "Yucca (Yucca gloriosa), Joshua-tree brevifolia." *Herbalist, II,* 1, 9-10, 1977.

28. Griffiths, G.J.: "Vaccine." *Reports on Chronic Rheum. Disease.* II, 56, 1936.

29. Harrington, H.D., "Y. Matsumura: Western Edible Wild Plants, Yucca." *Univ. of New Mexico Press,* 103-109, Albuquerque, 1972.

30. Herxheimer, Krause: "Eubereine Syphulitishen Vorkommende Quecksilberreaktion." *Dtsch. Med. Wchsch.,* 28:895-896, 1902.

31. Hoffman, J.: "Vaccine abstracts." *Soc. Amer. Bact.* N.Y. City Branch, Oct. 28. 1947.

32. Jaffe, Israeli A.: "Penicillamine." *Bull. on the Rheumatic Disease.* 28: 6, 948-953, 1977-78.

33. *J. Am Med. Assn.* "Editorial: Anti-arthritis drugs ranked for gastric-mucosal effect. 240:334, July 1978.

34. Jamison, A.; Anderson, K.: "Protozoa."
    Lancet, 1:261

35. Kingsburg, John M.: "Posisonous Plants of the
    United States and Canada." *Nightshades.*
    Prentice-Hall, N.J. 1968.

36. Kofoid, C.A., Swezy, O.: "Amebiasis of the
    bones." *(Protozoa)* J.A.M.A., 78: 1602-1604,
    1922.

37. *Lancet, Editorial:* "Pathogenic Free-Living
    Amoebae." 2: 165-166, 1977.

38. Livingstone Med. Clinic Personal Commun-
    cations. San Diego.

39. Marmor, L.; Warren, S.L.: "Ribonucleic acid
    particles in RA" *J. Rheum.* 6:2, 135-146, 1969.

40. Marmor, L.: "Surgery of Rheumatoid Arthri-
    tis." *Medical Treatment* 2:33 Lea & Febiger,
    Phildelphia, 1967.

41. Millman, M.: "An Allergic Concept of the Etio-
    logy of Rheumatoid Arthritis." *Ann. Allergy,*
    30:135-40, 1972.

42. Multicentre Study Group: "Levamisole in
    Rheumatoid Arthritis." *Lancet,* 2:1007-12, 1978.

43. McGuens, Jan: "A Review: Steroid Hormones
    and Plant Growth and Development." (Yucca)
    Phytochemistry, 17:1-14, 1978.

44. Nagington, J.; Watson, P.G.; Playfair, T.S. et al:
    "Amoebic Infection of the Eye." *Lancet* 2:1537-
    38, 1974.

45. Pearson, A.W.; Walsh, Michael J.: "Clinical
    Aspects of Nutrition in Rheumatic Fever." *J.
    Amer. Acad. Nutrition,* 1:102-109, 1947.

46. Pottinger, Francis M. Jr.: "The effect of heat processing foods on experimental animals." *Am. J. Orthodontia and Oral Surgery.*

47. Randolph, T.G.: "Ecologically Oriented Rheumatoid Arthritis." (In *"Clinical Ecology,"* Ed, Dickey.) Thomas, Springfield, Ohio, 1976.

48. Ridolfo, Anthony. "Non-steroidal Anti-inflammatory Agents in Arthritis." *American Family Practice.* Vol. 17: 2, 131-38. Feb. 1978.

49. Rowe, A.H.: "Food Allergy, Its Manifestations and Control with the Elimination Diets." *Thomas,* Springfield, 1972.

50. Sherwood, K.K.: "Vaccine for Arthritis" *N.W. Med.* 33:78, 1934.

51. Simon, S.W.; Renard, L.A.: "Vaccine." *Ann. Allergy,* 19: 877, Aug. 1961. And, 20: 175, March 1962. And, 25: 71, Sept. 1963.

52. Somers, Lowell H.: "A Retrospective Study of the Treatment of Rheumatoid Arthritis with Esterene." Sub. for pub. Mar. 20, 1980. Unpublished.

53. Spence, Patrick, F.: "Yucca, the Peanut of the Southwest." *East West,* 50-51, Dec. 1977.

54. Spencer, Michael: "Yucca, New Hope for Arthritics." *Let's Live,* 62-64, Feb. 1975.

55. Spielman, A.D.: "Vaccine." *N.Y. State J. of Med.* 55: 1603, June 1, 1955; *Arch. Otol.* 67:204, Feb. 1958.

56. Tew, J. et al: "Protozoa." *J. Immuno. Meth.* 14: 231, 1977.

57. Turnbull, J.A.,: "Study of 127 Cases of Arthritis." *Am. J. Dig. Dis.,* 11: 122-30, 1944.

58. Wall, M.E.; Eddy, C.R.; McClennon, M.L.; Klump, M.E.: "Detection and Estimation of Steroidal Sapogenin in Plant Tissue." (Yucca) *Analytical Chemistry* 24: 1337-41, 1952.

59. Webber, John M.: "Yuccas of the Southwest." *U.S. Dept. Agriculture,* Monograph No. 17. U. S. GPO, Washington, D.C., 1953.

60. Wilkins, Robert: "The use of non-steroidal anti-inflammatory agents." *JAMA,* 240: 1632-35, No. 15, Oct. 1978.

61. Wyatt, Bernard Langdon: "Nutrition in Arthritis." *J. Am. Acad. Applied Nutrition,* 1:88-91, 1947.

62. WYBURN-MASON, ROGER: "A New Protozoon: It's Relations to . . . Diseases." Kimpton, London, 1964.

"Protozoal Infection." *Pro. IX Int. Cong. Chemotherapy,* Plenum Press, N.Y. 1975.

"Rheumatoid Disease and Protozoa." Lancet, I:489, 1976.

"The Causation of Rheumatoid Disease, (etc.), a New Concept in Medicine." Iji Pub. Co., Tokyo, 1978.

"The Free-Living Amoebic Causation of Rheumatoid and Other Autoimmune Diseases." *Internal Medicine,* I:20-25, 1979.

"The Naeglerial Causation of Rheumatoid Disease (etc.) Medical Hypotheses," 5:1237-49, 1979.

"New Views on the Etiology of Rheumatoid Arthritis." *British Medicine,* 12-14, Aug. 21, 1979.

63. Yale, John W. Jr.: "Anti-Stress Properties of Steroid Saponins in Relation to Plant Growth." *Botanical Products Company,* Porterville, CA.

64. Yamagushi, K.: "Spectral Data of Natural Products, steroidal Sapogenins." (In Yucca) 1: 212-16, Elsevier Pub. Col, N.Y., 1970.

65. Zeller, M.: "Rheumatoid Arthritis, Food Allergy as a Factor." *Ann. Allergy,* 7:200-25, 1949.

66. Zussman, B.M.: "Food Hypersensitivity Simulating Rheumatoid Arthritis." *Southern Med. J.,* 59: 935-39, 1966.

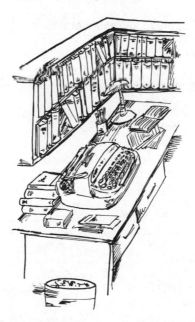

ARTHRITIS NEEDS COMMUNCIATION

INDEX

NOTE: The topics in capitals refer to chapter headings or subtitles They are found in the chapter which begins on the page given.

A

M

N